Dad

The ultimate guide to pregnancy, birth & dirty nappies

Dr Oscar Duke

Illustrations by Matt Chinworth

KYLE
BOOKS

For Rae and Rory, without whom there would be no story

An Hachette UK Company
www.hachette.co.uk

First published in Great Britain in 2019 by
Kyle Books, an imprint of Kyle Cathie Ltd
Carmelite House
50 Victoria Embankment
London EC4Y 0DZ
www.kylebooks.co.uk

Distributed in the US by Hachette Book Group,
1290 Avenue of the Americas, 4th and 5th Floors, New York, NY 10104.

Distributed in Canada by Canadian Manda Group, 664 Annette St., Toronto,
Ontario, Canada M6S 2C8.

ISBN: 978 085783 545 1

10 9 8 7 6 5 4 3 2 1

Publisher: Joanna Copestick
Illustrator: Matt Chinworth
Design: Dale Tomlinson
Project Editor: Sophie Allen
Production: Caroline Alberti

A Cataloguing in Publication record for this title is available from the British Library.

Printed and bound by CPI Group (UK) Ltd, Croydon, CR0 4YY

DISCLAIMER: The information and advice contained in this book are intended as
a general guide. Do not attempt self-diganosis or self-treatment for serious or long-term
conditions, including pregnancy, before consulting a medical professional or qualified
practitioner. This book is not intended to be a substitute for taking proper medical advice
and should not be relied upon in any way. The author and publisher cannot accept
responsibility for illness arising out of the failure to seek medical advice from a doctor.

Contents

Introduction

I've spent years looking after pregnant women and supporting parents as they welcome their new arrivals into the world. Watching as they scramble to care for them in the best possible way, without dropping them, allowing them to vomit on unsuspecting friends or cover too many carpets with bright yellow poo.

As a doctor, you might have thought that after all the hours of studying, night shifts and exams I'd taken, that I'd know it all, but really I felt like a fraud. Deep down I knew that there'd be no substitute for the first-hand experience of becoming a dad myself — and I wasn't wrong. Within a week of having my daughter, I'd learnt more useful and practical information about how to care for a baby than any textbook, on-call shift or antenatal class could ever have taught me.

The greatest surprise for me was the vast range of different emotions I felt as the process of becoming a parent so quickly unfolded before my eyes. None of the books I'd come across addressed how a dad might feel as he discovered he was having a baby or stood by watching as his child's head appeared from the entrance of a vagina. Some of these are elating, some terrifying and others just mind-blowing. But with alarmingly increasing rates of post-natal anxiety and depression amongst new dads, I felt these conversations needed to be had.

Understanding the facts gives you some armour, but I hope that by sharing my personal experiences and those of many of my patients, this book will equip you mentally to cope with all that lies ahead as you discover, in your own way, how to be a dad.

Baby growth chart

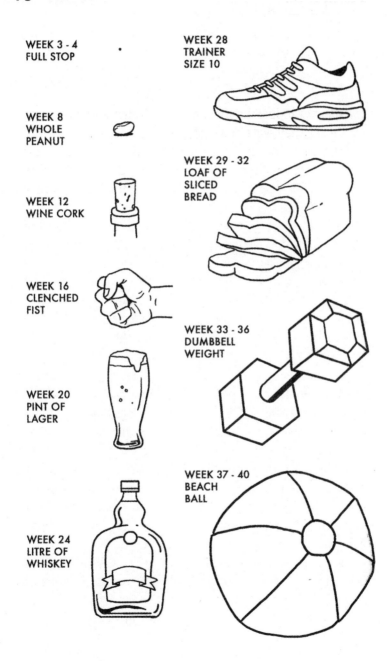

WEEK 3 - 4
FULL STOP

WEEK 8
WHOLE
PEANUT

WEEK 12
WINE CORK

WEEK 16
CLENCHED
FIST

WEEK 20
PINT OF
LAGER

WEEK 24
LITRE OF
WHISKEY

WEEK 28
TRAINER
SIZE 10

WEEK 29 - 32
LOAF OF
SLICED
BREAD

WEEK 33 - 36
DUMBBELL
WEIGHT

WEEK 37 - 40
BEACH
BALL

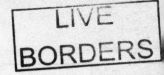

1

Balls

Where it all begins

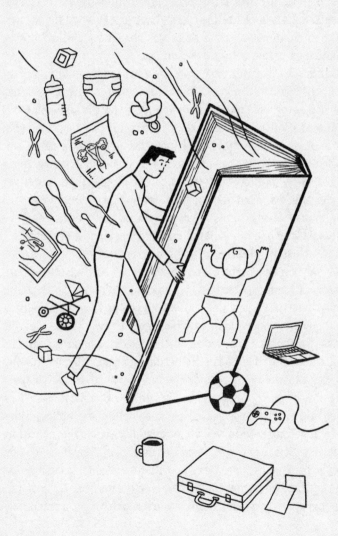

FROM THE DOCTOR

Ever since you burst onto the planet, these two little, or not so little, reservoirs of life have been there. Often in the way, liable to painful injury (and hidden away from your mum at the earliest sight of a pubic hair), these potential life-givers – which, if you've listened to health advice, you might have occasionally checked for lumps and bumps – are now at the forefront of your mind. You may have picked up this book because yours have just excelled themselves in their child-making class or simply because you're wondering about their potential for future success.

After years of 'getting it on before you get it off' or enquiring cautiously as to whether your partner has remembered her particular form of contraception that day, now the game plan has changed. If you're anything like me, the fear of catching chlamydia or another sexually transmitted infection has always paled into insignificance beside the prospect of an unintentional pregnancy. We all know that most infections can be either cured or treated highly effectively, but the thought of becoming a dad is, quite simply, on another level. This is a game-changer that begins the very moment your balls do their life-creating thing for the first time.

Women have libraries of books, blogs, podcasts and magazines that devote billions of pages to the experience of conception, pregnancy and childbirth. By writing this I in no way intended to undermine the huge physical, psychological and hormonal journey that any pregnant woman goes through. However, I hope that this book, written as it is by a doctor who has cast aside the condoms and ridden the rollercoaster to becoming a dad, will go some way towards answering those 'man questions' that never quite make it to pubs, locker-rooms, water coolers or any other locations where men might find themselves having meaningful chats. Although let's face it, getting men to talk about anything personal is almost as difficult as it is to get an egg fertilized by a sperm. Hopefully reading this will give you a head start when it comes to understanding what the hell is going on now that a baby is on the horizon. Think of it as a papery man-hug that can guide you through what is a potentially treacherous world of terminology, hormones, social change, sleep deprivation and finally dirty nappies with tiny feet attached.

Learning the basics

In my fourth year at medical school, after years of studying biochemistry, hearts, lungs, bones and all the organs in between, the syllabus finally turned to obstetrics, the branch of medicine responsible for helping women to grow babies and bring them into the world. I really couldn't have been less interested in the subject. Granted, this was before the days of *One Born Every Minute* being on the TV, so just seeing a freshly birthed baby spring through its mother's legs or being removed from her open abdomen was pretty novel, but the thought of having a child of my own was completely off my radar. In the first week we underwent the most bizarre and by now legendary element of medical training to date – well beyond the realms of dissecting preserved human bodies. We were split into small groups to meet the Gynaecology Teaching Associates, a pair of delightful middle-aged women who taught us, by live demonstration on each other, how to perform a vaginal examination and how to use a speculum (the notorious plastic duck-beak-shaped implement dreaded by women having smear tests) to look through the vagina to see the cervix, the gateway to the womb, or uterus. One by one we joined a queue to practise while the lady in question gave feedback, the content of which is etched on my mind forever: 'Very good, now just take your thumb off my clitoris' or, 'Perfectly done, just try not to catch a pube next time'. Well, how else were we supposed to learn? The cervix is going to feature heavily in this story. You might have felt it if you've ever put anything with sensation inside a vagina. It feels a bit like the tip of your nose and looks like a very small doughnut – round with a tiny hole in the middle. Some say it actually just looks like the head of a penis staring at you from the back of the vagina.

Several years later, as a fully qualified junior doctor working in a sexual health clinic, I began my first professional search for a woman's cervix. As the woman climbed onto the examination couch, she asked if it mattered that she was on her period. It didn't, so I politely reassured her that there was no need to worry – this was true for her, but not for me. A tiny bit of my inner man cringed. I had a flashback to GCSE biology, and those complicated graphs you might remember showing the hormonal changes of the menstrual cycle. But my real fear was of the period blood itself and stick with me here. As soon as I saw it, my perception changed forever: this was not the stuff of horror films, this blood was a gentle trickle, neatly oozing from the opening of the cervix and flowing into the vagina, a remarkable, natural phenomenon that's a sign of fertility and of life to come. Just for a moment I felt like David Attenborough, marvelling over the natural world. I briefly contemplated a breathy voice-over but remembered myself, took a quick swab and withdrew the speculum. I had escaped unharmed.

The baby-making

So after years of irrational period 'man fear', and the relief that the contraception had yet again done us proud, my attention now turned to a completely opposite aim – baby-making. A world where the sight of vaginal blood is more unwanted than ever before. You may have arrived here after battling through months of ovulation calculators, period apps and militant sex schedules. Perhaps you've finally succeeded with some help from a fertility clinic, or have accidentally got somebody pregnant and are now wondering, with shrinking testicles, what might lie ahead.

A few generations back, men provided the sperm, paid for all the baby gear and went straight back to work. Before that, and you've seen the period dramas, men just jumped on, did the business until they'd satisfied themselves and moved on. In every way that it's right relationships have changed and developed since those days, it's also right that men, indeed dads, should expect to understand and fully participate in the making, growing, birthing and parenting of their children. Obviously, you can uncross your legs, you're not going to hurt downstairs but being an informed, involved father can improve pregnancy outcomes, as well as childhood behaviour and relationships for years to come. And no, this doesn't just depend on whether or not you do the washing-up. Modern relationships are, luckily for men and women, farting in the face of stereotype.

From stay-at-home dads to same-sex parents, industry-leading mums, to full-time mannies, never has the role of dad been so varied. Whichever one you find yourself contemplating, fatherhood will bring its own huge rewards and challenges.

You may be asking yourself: When is the right time to have a child? How will it affect my life, relationship, job or family? Can I afford it? These are all very sensible questions, which certainly ran through my mind when I finally agreed to let the sperm flow freely in the rampant – you should have seen the schedule – quest for fatherhood. My wife had wanted children since time began and this feeling had certainly intensified since we had married – the best men even mentioned the prospect of children in their speech. But what did I want? I knew I did, one day, want to be a dad, but when? Is now right, I thought? Am I grown up enough? I was recently asked for ID when trying to buy a bottle of Sauvignon in the supermarket. 'I'm 31', I replied. 'But you look so young,' said the sales assistant, as if this was some sort of compliment – before he refused to accept my NHS ID card, which clearly stated that I was a doctor, as evidence for me meeting the legal drinking age. Medically, we now know that a man's sperm deteriorates in quality as he ages, which may bring with it an increased risk of conditions such as autism in your child. It's not exactly the ticking time bomb of female fertility, but worth a thought as research reveals more. In reality though, there probably never is a perfect time. In my situation a quick check of the job status revealed I was likely to be employed for a while, our relationship seemed wonderful and the balls were producing something, but who knew whether it contained anything worthwhile?

I obviously can't look into the unique situation of every potential dad-to-be in this tome, but whatever your concerns are, rest assured, there is always help and advice available. In my case, I had a fear of passing on the genetic condition albinism (a pigment disorder resulting in white hair and skin and a severe visual impairment) that I live with every day. While it's not a life-limiting condition, it's still pretty undesirable. I might have felt differently about it if somebody had told me they were casting people with albinism in *The Da Vinci Code* or that Harry Potter's nemesis Draco

Malfoy was in fact ridiculously blond, but I knew I'd prefer to pass some of my better qualities on to a child and not curse them with a life of peering at screens and being unable to work out which bus is about to run them over. So, I went to see a geneticist. After a painstaking wait, my inbuilt error was finally identified. A tiny, but significant, faulty gene in my DNA – talk about scrutinizing yourself. I was told that I'd pass the gene to all my offspring (horrible word), but they'd only have albinism if my wife carried the gene too. She's not albino, we're not related (as far as we know), so we decided to leave it to chance. Unnervingly though, I realized I'd just bought a lottery ticket, so I must in some way believe in small chances winning through. As I have recently made a TV documentary about the murder and mutilation of people with albinism in East Africa, my perceptions have somewhat changed. Albinism is certainly not ideal, but worse things could happen. I'll uncover the mysteries of routine genetic screening during pregnancy later in the book.

This brings us neatly back to my balls, or yours for that matter. Exactly half of your genetic make-up is neatly packaged into each tiny sperm. All being well, during ejaculation more than 39 million sperm, suspended in nutrient-rich seminal fluid, leave your penis travelling at over 20mph. The volume varies, but on average 3.7ml (approximately three quarters of a teaspoon) of the little swimmers head out on a challenging, perilous journey that few survive. Fortunately for us men, the chances of surviving the journey ahead are far greater, so ready the balls and let the voyage to fatherhood begin.

FROM THE DAD

Being a doctor allows me to explain all the factual elements of this exciting journey into fatherhood in a way that I hope is both interesting and understandable to someone with no medical training. But the science, procedures and jargon that I've picked up throughout my training and career are only a tiny fraction of what I've had to learn as I've become a dad myself. So, I've added a 'From the Dad' section to each chapter, providing an insight into how I, and the hundreds of dads that I've met, both professionally and personally, think and feel as we embark on one of life's biggest and greatest challenges. It's an emotional process so you may as well hear it as it is from guys who've been there before. No two men will ever have the same experience and yours will be completely unique, too. If you are at the start of the adventure, however you do or don't define your gender or sexuality and in whatever capacity you've come to be considering fatherhood, I hope this book will go some way towards facilitating and enhancing your experience.

What Women Want

While dads can take many roles along this journey, so far, the one thing we can't do is grow and carry a baby. But you can be an invaluable source of support for your partner. So, at the end of each chapter there's a box featuring the top **DO**s and **DON'T**s for dads-to-be from a survey of pregnant women I've conducted, telling you in their own words how you can help ease the burden for your partner. It seems only fair!

2

Uterus

From fertility to foetus

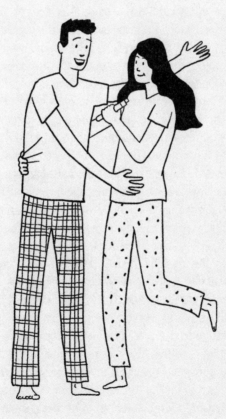

FROM THE DOCTOR

Maybe years of planning have now resulted in your partner thinking she's pregnant or perhaps you've received a terrifying phone call from a woman telling you she's missed her period. Either way, stay calm, breathe and get a pregnancy test to confirm things officially. Your partner can buy a home-testing kit from any pharmacy or supermarket or go to her doctor or a sexual health clinic.

When your super-swimming sperm combines with its now inseparable egg friend, it makes its way down a fallopian tube (the fine pipes that connect the ovaries to the uterus) and embeds itself in the wall of the uterus. As it develops, the placenta – the alien-like object that acts as a buffet for the baby to provide a constant supply of perfectly prepared food throughout pregnancy – begins to form and implants itself into the wall of the uterus and releases a hormone called human chorionic gonadotropin (or hCG) into the blood stream. Blood is filtered by the kidneys and this hCG passes into the woman's urine. This so-called 'implantation' can happen any time between 6 and 12 days after an egg is released by the ovaries (ovulation). Whatever the promises made on the packaging, pregnancy test kits all work in pretty much the same way. Whether your partner collects the urine in a pot and dips the stick into it or pees directly onto the stick, the presence of hCG is what gives the positive result. Different kits claim to detect pregnancy at different stages; some even guarantee to pick it up a week before a missed period. This is all marvellous stuff. If you're anything like other expectant parents, you'll probably have spent a small fortune on overpriced test kits before you're satisfied that the thin blue positive lines are not just a figment of your imagination. However, even a faint line means the test is positive and confirms that the 'bun' is well and truly in the 'oven'. If the test isn't positive and there's still no sign of that period, give it a few days and try again; most kits come with at least two test sticks anyway.

Before you spread the news

Instead of rushing out to shout from the rooftops or fill social media with images of your wee-soaked test sticks, it's worth spending just a few miserable minutes thinking about some of the possible things that can go wrong in the early days of pregnancy. Occasionally, the sperm–egg combo fails to implant in the correct place in the uterus and instead gets stuck outside of the uterus, for example in a fallopian tube. This is known as an ectopic pregnancy and not only will the baby sadly not survive, but if unspotted it can pose a huge danger to your partner so it needs to be removed. This can either be done by taking medication or by undergoing a surgical procedure. Only about 12,000 ectopic pregnancies occur in the UK each year. Signs to look out for include vaginal bleeding, tummy pain or, weirdly, pain in the tip of the shoulder. To confuse things further, a small amount of bleeding can occur normally during implantation, even when everything's going well. So, to be on the safe side, discuss any bleeding or tummy pain that occurs in pregnancy with your doctor or midwife, who can arrange a scan if they're concerned to see exactly what's going on in there.

While we're talking about bleeding in early pregnancy, it's worth remembering that this could also be a sign of miscarriage. About one in four known pregnancies end in miscarriage, but it's thought many more may have occurred before a woman even realizes she's pregnant. Miscarriage is often the result of an underlying genetic problem with the growing baby and most - around 85 per cent - occur within the first 12 weeks of pregnancy. Undoubtedly this is a very difficult and upsetting experience for both you and your partner to find yourselves in, but remember that there is a lot of support available. Importantly, most miscarriages are one-offs and the majority of women go on to have successful pregnancies in the future. Being told that these events are very common can seem little consolation at the time but try to keep positive, embrace the support and, when you and your partner feel emotionally and physically ready, get those sperm swimming again.

How long is a pregnancy?

Now let's get back to the mini-you now safely nestled in your partner's uterus. Pregnancy is all about the timeline and it's worth even the most disorganized dad-to-be getting his head around this at an early stage. The 'nine months' of pregnancy so often talked about is really 40 weeks of 'gestation', which the more mathematically minded will realize isn't really nine months at all. The pregnancy timeline is traditionally broken down into three parts, episodes or seasons known as 'trimesters'. The first trimester takes you up to week 13, the second runs from weeks 14 to 27 and the third from week 28 to the big delivery day itself. And while 40 weeks is the magic number, remember that it's completely normal for a woman to give birth at any time between weeks 37 and 42 and have what's known as a 'term baby'. This is a baby that, as far as us medical types are concerned, is born at a normal and safe time, and all being well would be expected to survive without medical assistance in the big wide world – obviously, they will need some help though, so don't stop reading just yet.

As the months stretch out before you, you'll probably be frantically trying to calculate when your baby is 'due' to arrive. Now here's a calculation nobody covered in the maths class. Pregnancy lasts 40 weeks, but from when? You might be pretty sure of the night, day or even lazy afternoon that Mummy met Daddy and conception occurred, but even if you log your sex schedule on your smart-phone calendar, you're unlikely to be able to work out the exact day of conception. This is because sperm can survive for up to 7 days once they've made their way into the friendly female reproductive tract and even if your partner has her day of ovulation tattooed onto her, an egg can also survive at least a day before conception occurs. So, to make the calculation a little easier, the 'estimated delivery date' (or EDD) is calculated as 40 weeks from the first day of your partner's last period. And the key is in the 'E' – this is very much an estimate. Some women, particularly those with irregular periods, will struggle to calculate the exact date. A baby's birth is not like a microwave that's suddenly going to start beeping and fling the door open as soon as the set time is reached. Babies have a habit of arriving when they're ready, but the EDD is at least a rough guide that helps with all the planning that lies ahead. Sorry, but it's all we can offer at the moment. If you're currently scrolling through your calendar and losing count, a shortcut formula might help: identify the first day of the last period, go back 3 months, then add on 7 days and you get the due date. Alternatively, make life really easy and use one of the many EDD calculators available online.

Staying healthy really helps

Whenever I first meet a woman who's just discovered she's pregnant, the conversation inevitably turns to what she should and shouldn't be doing to protect her unborn baby's health as the trimesters meander by. It's hard not to sound like a nutritionist life coach when dispensing advice to dads-to-be too, but the essence is pretty simple: keeping your partner healthy will also keep your baby healthy. Your partner should avoid all of the things we secretly already know are bad for us, but there are a few pregnancy extras.

But before she starts giving things up, there are two things to add in straight away. Folic acid supplements protect against neural-tube defects, such as spina bifida, and should be ideally started 12 weeks prior to conception and continued at least until the 12th week of pregnancy. Most women will need to take 400 micrograms of folic acid each day. But women who are overweight (BMI >30), or suffer from diabetes or coeliac disease, or who are on certain epilepsy medications, will need a higher dose so need to seek specialist advice. A daily supplement of vitamin D is also recommended for all pregnant and breastfeeding women. Handily, plenty of companies have combined these two supplements into a daily pregnancy pill.

One thing that has to go, without doubt, is smoking. Everybody's agreed that smoking causes significant harm to both mum and baby, and increases the risk of ectopic pregnancy, miscarriage and stillbirth. If your partner's a smoker, the healthcare team will offer extensive support to help her give up, and normally undertake carbon-monoxide breath testing – it's a bit like an alcohol breathalyzer – to confirm that she's stopped. Kicking the habit can be tricky, but there's never been a better excuse and people are three times more likely to give up smoking with support from a professional and some form of nicotine replacement therapy. So, embrace the gum, patches and lozenges – all of which are safe in pregnancy.

Even if your partner doesn't smoke, being around people who smoke is harmful to your baby, so if you or anybody else you live with is still puffing away, now's the time to get responsible and kick the habit too for the sake of your unborn child. Passive smoking is linked to stillbirth and sudden infant death syndrome (SIDS), or cot death (see Chapter 17), as well as hampering baby's growth and health. And no, before you ask, having a cheeky fag out of the window isn't going to solve the problem I'm afraid. Traces of toxic chemicals on clothes and around the home environment are where all the problems begin. Hard as it might be, smoking has to go!

Alcohol is always a subject of much debate. Many an expectant dad panics that his partner had been drinking alcohol before she knew she was pregnant. This is a waste of time. Firstly, there's nothing you can now do to remove those glasses of wine or even that bottle of prosecco knocked back at the office party and secondly, it's very unlikely to have caused any significant problems. That said, once you know she's pregnant, the official advice is that your partner should avoid all alcohol throughout pregnancy. Drinking alcohol, especially during the first trimester, can increase the risk of miscarriage and premature birth and excessive intake can lead to foetal alcohol syndrome. Some pregnant women do choose to have the occasional alcoholic drink, but keeping intake to a minimum is important.

Although 'eating for two' isn't a thing, it's worth helping your partner out with some of the dos and don'ts of healthy eating for pregnancy lifestyle – healthy mum = healthy baby. There are some foods that should be avoided altogether as they carry a higher risk of infections that may either upset mum or potentially cause damage to your unborn baby. Let's begin with cheese. The first rule is no cheese made with unpasteurized milk. Beyond that, hard cheeses are all good. Mould-ripened, stinky soft cheeses like Brie, Camembert, blue cheeses and some goat's cheeses have a small risk of infecting mum and baby with listeria, an infection known as listeriosis that can cause birth defects or miscarriage. But cheese lovers relax; this risk is massively reduced if the cheese is cooked. So, bake a camembert, pop the blue cheese on a pizza or grill some goat's cheese and whack it in a salad. Soft processed cheeses like mozzarella, feta and ricotta made from pasteurized milk are perfectly safe. I'm a doctor, not a chef, but a little bit of culinary genius can suddenly make the pregnancy restrictions look a whole lot less bleak.

While we're in the kitchen, raw or uncooked meats carry the risk of infection with toxoplasmosis – a parasite also found in cat poo and unpasteurized goat's milk. (Not even a chef could successfully combine those two ingredients into an attractive menu option.) So, cook meat thoroughly and if your partner's desperate for a platter of uncooked or cured meats like salami or prosciutto, either freeze them for 4 days first to kill those nasty parasites or scatter them over that pizza you've already covered with stinking ripe cheese and pop it in the oven.

On the subject of freezing, restrictions have now relaxed about eating raw fish; sushi lovers can still indulge as long as the fish has been frozen beforehand. However, a pregnant woman should avoid shark, swordfish or marlin as they contain high levels of mercury that may damage baby's nervous system. She should also not eat more than two tuna steaks per week or four medium sized cans of tinned tuna because of its mercury levels. The advice is to avoid excess oily fish too – that's things like salmon, mackerel, herring and trout; keep to no more than two portions a week. Finally, while we're going nuts in the food cupboard, we'd best talk about peanuts. There's currently no evidence that eating peanuts during pregnancy increases the risk of peanut allergy in children, so despite what you might hear, if she loves peanuts, who are we to argue?

FROM THE DAD

We hadn't been trying for a baby for long when a few night shifts got in the way of what my wife considered to be 'proper trying'; there's nothing quite like a night on call to kill the libido. A combination of apps, ovulation detectors and abandoned contraception meant that my wife, a self-professed non-scientist, was now behaving like a professor of fertility medicine. As the usual period date approached, excitement soared. Could this be it? Had we done it at the first attempt? The message came through at work the following day accompanied by a string of sad-faced emojis. The period had come, and no, we weren't quite the fertile superhumans we'd somehow hoped we might be. There was definite criticism of my sperm - probably their fault - and a school-report-style feedback note of 'must try harder'.

So, sparing you the further specific details, it wasn't long before there really was no period. A week passed and still nothing; after two weeks, the temptation to test became unbearable, so with a new job about to start the following day, we bought the pregnancy test kits and off she went to do the business. I'd previously laughed at the ridiculous TV adverts for pregnancy test kits, where a delighted woman with tears of joy in her eyes comes out of the bathroom brandishing a wee-soaked stick with two little blue positive lines on it. But suddenly here I was, confronted by exactly that. A sense of disbelief, a desire to buy all the kits and test again and again, the joy of success and the fear of not being up to the job of dad. In that instant I went from a doctor with all the theoretical knowledge of pregnancy, birth and parenting, to a dad-to-be with the realization that I lacked all the practical experience of what it truly meant to be a father. It turns out the flood of emotions I felt in that moment was not unusual. Despite this being a planned pregnancy, I couldn't stop questioning whether now was really the right time. Were we really up to the job and how much would our lives have to change? All of this was superficial worry though compared to the underlying warm glow that was flowing through my veins. An amazing sense of pride and joy. I was going to be a dad and, ready or not, this baby was coming for me. I vowed there and then to embrace and enjoy whatever journey lay ahead.

For another dad-to-be, things weren't going quite so smoothly. The delight of a positive pregnancy test was followed by an evening spent in the local emergency department with his partner having cramping pains and vaginal bleeding. The doctors felt it wasn't an ectopic pregnancy, but warned it may be the signs of miscarriage and asked them to return the following day for a scan. He described his horror as the lovely nurse performing the scan raised a dildo-style ultrasound probe and covered it with what appeared to be a condom, before adding a bit of lubrication and inserting it into his partner's vagina. The scan was painless for his partner, but for both of them, the wait seemed interminable. Within seconds however, uninterpretable images were appearing on the nearby monitor and it wasn't long before they were reassured that a live, 'viable' pregnancy was seen, along with a foetal heartbeat. The sense of relief in the room was immense. It was a first look into the anxieties parenthood can bring and a stark reminder that dads-to-be are going to need to get used to things becoming a bit clinical in the vagina department.

Not spreading the news!

Trying to keep the exciting pregnancy news from friends and family for the first few weeks was far more difficult than I'd ever imagined, mainly because of my difficulty in keeping a poker face and the sudden onslaught of events where my wife would normally have been drinking alcohol. I soon became the master of a solo visit to the bar to secretly request drinks that would pass for alcohol but not cause any damage to the bundle of cells now growing at an alarming rate inside the uterus. Soda water dressed up as a Gin & Tonic does the trick perfectly. My wife turned down several invitations to events where she thought friends might guess what was going on, but started to feel a bit isolated by the secret. Eating out suddenly became a challenge too. Why was she suddenly so against goat's cheese and what was our new-found interrogation of waiters at sushi restaurants all about?

Traditionally couples wait until the 12-week dating scan before announcing their news, but it's got to be a personal decision that's right for you. Another dad told me he didn't see the point in waiting to tell people. Well aware that things could go wrong in the early days, he and his partner had decided that even if they did have problems, they'd want the support of their nearest and dearest, so why not involve them from the outset? Whichever way you go, choose carefully who you decide to share the early news with and, if you're taking the secret approach, support your partner through the difficult months as your friends and family wonder why you've gone slightly under the radar or developed some crazy new lifestyle habits. In reality, they'll probably be on to you, so all-out denial seems to be a pretty good policy to adopt too.

What Women Want

DO be strong, supportive and don't panic – it's amazing and terrifying at the same time for both of you.

DON'T run through every alcoholic drink or piece of cheese your partner consumed in the last month before the positive pregnancy test and panic about the potential damage done.

3

Brain

Mind, midwives and the first trimester

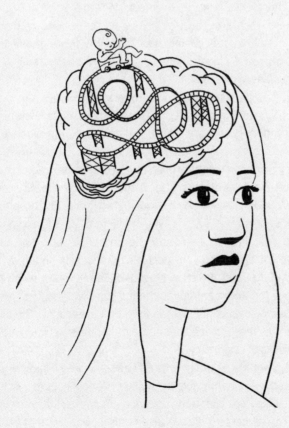

FROM THE DOCTOR

As the first trimester gets underway, pregnancy hormones are racing through the body. Surging blood levels of oestrogen and progesterone are often accompanied by mood changes and a rollercoaster of emotions. Most women notice the psychological impact of these changes between weeks six and ten of pregnancy and often even surprise themselves at how dramatic and unprovoked their mood swings can be. The good news is that things normally settle down as the friendly second trimester approaches, so hold tight and quietly remember that it's probably just the hormones and their effects on the brain's neuro-transmitters that are causing what can seem like irrational behaviour. Uphold the golden rule though – never make the mistake of reassuringly blaming her hormonal state; this inevitably leads to disaster.

While your partner's hormonal rollercoaster loops the loop and your baby's doing some of their most important development of the pregnancy, you are probably left wondering when the healthcare professionals start to be involved. If the positive pregnancy test hasn't already been flicked under the nose of your doctor, you should contact your local antenatal or maternity care team at around the six-week mark. All midwife units and hospitals now offer a self-referral system – you can generally book in without bothering your doctor. There may be an online form for your partner to complete and your doctor's practice will be happy to point you in the right direction if needed. Either way, it won't be long before the antenatal appointments start winging their way into the diary – expect at least ten for a first pregnancy. The first one, known as the 'booking appointment', happens between eight and ten weeks of pregnancy.

Now appointments mean time off work and we all know what that can cause – unhappy bosses, managers or colleagues – so it's worth knowing both your and your partner's rights. Starting with the baby carrier herself – if she's an employee, whether that's full- or part-time, under UK law she's entitled to 'reasonable' time off to attend antenatal appointments, without losing any pay. These can be for any routine part of antenatal care or any other classes advised or recommended by a midwife or doctor. Dads, sadly, don't quite get the same deal as their partner. They are entitled to time off to attend two antenatal appointments, but whether or not this is paid is at the discretion of their employer. As with all employment benefits, it's important to check your and your partner's contracts carefully for specific benefits and don't leave it too late to tell your employer the news.

Question, questions...

Your booking appointment is the first opportunity for you and your partner to meet the healthcare professionals – midwives and doctors – who will be involved in caring for your partner and baby during pregnancy. It's the ideal time to ask all those burning questions you've both been chewing over as you desperately attempt to avoid goat's cheese, raw meat and suspicious friends or family. It's not a one-way process though. The midwife will also have what seems like an unending list of questions for your partner – and you. The purpose of this is to identify medical, psychological or even social issues that may impact on either mum or baby as the pregnancy progresses. So, ensure your partner is ready to talk about any medical conditions, ongoing medications, previous pregnancies, miscarriages, terminations or other factors that might be important for the team to know. They'll want to know about disorders that may run in the family (genetic disorders) – hers and yours – and ask about infections, such as HIV or hepatitis. Don't be shocked. There's no judgement at work here, it's just standard information that needs to be checked to ensure the safe arrival of baby-you. Couples often ask if they need to disclose everything or whether they can keep an event like a previous termination private. Sharing as much information as you can, as openly as possible, will mean your partner and baby can receive the best available care.

If you're accompanying your partner to the booking appointment, don't be offended if you're asked to leave the room for a period of time while the midwife speaks to your partner alone. Again, this is a normal procedure to allow her time to disclose any information she may not feel comfortable discussing in front of you. This can feel pretty weird and many dads-to-be find it a bit of a negative experience, especially if they feel their relationship is exceptionally honest and open. Just go with the flow and reassure yourself that it's all part of the procedure. It's not a police interview and it isn't something for anyone to fear.

Aside from medical conditions and medications, the team will also want to know about any mental health problems that your partner either currently experiences or has had in the past. Pregnancy is a stressful time both physically and emotionally and luckily these days, as healthcare professionals, we're interested in caring for the whole mum-to-be, not just her bump. Conditions such as depression and anxiety can worsen during pregnancy or even be identified for the very first time, so a good understanding of any pre-existing conditions is vital and enables appropriate support to be offered early. Some women have significant phobias surrounding pregnancy and delivery of babies and, if that's the case for your partner, encourage her to flag this at an early stage. Obviously, the thought of carrying and having a baby brings a level of anxiety for both parents. Being pregnant and getting the baby out – however it's done – is no walk in the park, so some anxiety and even fear is completely normal. Expectant mums with heightened levels of fear or anxiety may be suffering from a condition known as tocophobia, or the fear of giving birth, which affects 6–10 per cent of women. It can be caused by a previous traumatic birth experience, but can also exist in first-time mums. Airing any such concerns as soon as possible means that early support and birth planning can be put in place to enable your partner to enjoy her pregnancy without unnecessary anxiety.

No matter how relaxed (or not) you're both feeling about the pregnancy, once the midwives have finished their questioning, now's your chance to clarify any areas of what lies ahead that need further explanation. Much better to hear it from a seasoned pro than a web-based forum full of rumours and hearsay, so it's a good idea to prepare a list of any questions you might have before your visit. Otherwise, inevitably you arrive full of things you both want to know and by the time the opportunity comes to ask questions, they've left your head completely or your partner's too busy freaking out about the forthcoming blood tests to remember what it was she really wanted to know.

You'll also be given information about locally available antenatal classes. These won't start until much later in pregnancy, but it's a good opportunity to work out what's on offer and get booked in, as whether they're run by the hospital, clinic or a private organization, these can be invaluable. Attending together is a brilliant idea, and once you've read this book, you'll be close to top of the class before you even start. Geek!

What are the tests about?

Inevitably there will be some blood tests needed at the outset, so be ready for the supportive hand-hold if your partner's squeamish, and if it's you who's more likely to collapse at the sight of blood, keep your eyes on her and avoid the needle and sample bottles. Testing is done for anaemia (a low red blood cell count often caused by iron deficiency), kidney and liver function, infections like HIV and hepatitis as well as genetic disorders like sickle cell disease. Your partner's blood group will also be identified. This is important for two reasons. First, the hospital will need to know which blood type to offer your partner if she experiences heavy bleeding during labour or delivery and needs a blood transfusion. Secondly, and way more complicated, the 'rhesus status' of mum's blood needs to be checked too. Now what on earth is that all about? Hold tight there Dad, biology lesson coming right at you.

Most of the cells in our body carry small markers called antigens that poke out from their surface. These antigens allow the cells to be identified as either friends or enemies by other cells in the body. Some people's red blood cells carry a D antigen, making them rhesus-D positive; some have no such antigen and they are said to be rhesus-D negative. It's all determined by our genes and there's nothing we can do to change it. If your partner's red blood cells are rhesus-D positive, there's nothing further to worry about. Science lesson over. If, however, her blood is rhesus-D negative, and carries no D antigen, you'll be staying for an extra science class. What happens next is determined by you. If your red blood cells carry the D antigen, it may have been passed on to your baby in your genes. When a rhesus-D negative mother carries a rhesus-D positive baby, things get a little more complex. If the baby's blood is exposed to the mother's blood during labour, delivery or at any other time during the pregnancy, the mother's blood may produce cells called antibodies to fight off the unfamiliar D antigens from baby's blood. This isn't usually a problem for the first pregnancy, but once these antibodies exist they lurk in the mother's blood and may attack a baby's red blood cells during future pregnancies, destroying baby's red blood cells and causing potentially dangerous anaemias. So, to prevent this, a rhesus-negative mother will be offered an injection of 'Anti-D' at 28 weeks of pregnancy and at any other points in the pregnancy where bleeding may have occurred. After the birth, the baby's blood will be checked and if it's found to be rhesus-D positive, a further injection of 'Anti-D' will be given to mum to prevent issues in subsequent pregnancies.

Now if you're not an expert in the immune system and have grasped even a flavour of what's happening here, congratulations. It's normally something I have to read several times before it finally begins to make sense – even in my medical mind. So, there's absolutely no shame in re-reading the paragraph until the full sci-fi-like plot of the battle between antibodies and rhesus D is clear in your mind too. If you're still none the wiser, in summary: rhesus-positive mum – no issue; rhesus-negative mums will normally need 'Anti-D' injections to protect future babies against blood disorders. Lesson complete.

What lies ahead?

At your booking visit your partner will be given a personal maternity record book, which the healthcare team will use to enter her medical notes for the entire pregnancy – and wherever she goes, so too should these notes. As long as she gives you permission to do so, I'd recommend both of you having a good read. The book contains a lot of really useful information about the services available in your area and how processes work at your local hospital, as well as contact numbers for pregnancy-related emergencies. Make sure you know where they're kept and that your partner takes them with her when she's away from home. The record book should be taken to all medical appointments, but should also be near at hand if your partner suddenly needs help when away from home, at work or on holiday. The notes will be invaluable to doctors and midwives if you suddenly pitch up in a clinic or hospital that hasn't previously been providing care for your partner. More importantly even than this, if she rocks up to appointments without the notes, the look she might receive from an unimpressed midwife may traumatize you both for several years to come. You have been warned!

The record book will include a care schedule listing the timings for future scans and appointments. You will also be given advice on the options for your care and the type of delivery your partner wants (more on this in Chapter 10). Your care options vary from area to area but typically, this will be a combination of visits to the midwife or your doctor during the weeks that follow. There may be appointments with specialist consultants if there are any complications with either your partner or baby's health. For an uncomplicated first pregnancy, your partner might expect to attend around ten different appointments, and more if closer monitoring is required; a second pregnancy will routinely have seven. The first dating scan is usually performed around 12 weeks and a further, more detailed, 'anomaly scan' is carried out at around 20 weeks. (More on these later in Chapters 5 and 8). All other visits will involve a check-up for mum and baby, with monitoring of your partner's blood pressure, a urine test and a feel and measure of baby in the ever-expanding tummy. But fear not. All will be explained in due course.

FROM THE DAD

It turns out that the rumours about crazy pregnancy-related mood changes are completely true. In the eight years I'd known her prior to becoming pregnant, my wife had never, in any way, been physically aggressive towards me - or anybody else for that matter. Now I'm only sharing this story in the interests of transparency and, of course, by the time you're reading this my punishment will probably mean I'm about as far away from any future fathering as a man with a vasectomy, but things changed dramatically one evening during the first trimester. Undoubtedly provoked by a careless comment from me, I suddenly found myself to be the victim of a crockery attack. I'm told the china bowl wasn't thrown at me, just near me, but it certainly made some pretty smashing contact with the very same piece of kitchen floor I was standing on. I'm ashamed to say I responded appallingly. Shocked by what had just happened, I walked out, and both of us were in tears. Let me emphasize though that nothing like this has ever happened before (or since). A few minutes later, with a cooler head, I reflected on what had happened, reminded myself that this was not just my wife, but also a pregnant woman, carrying my child. I pulled myself together, returned home and made up while we debated who would order the replacement bowl online.

I was pleased to discover we are not the only people this has happened to, with other parents I've spoken to telling me of pieces of, weirdly, crockery that have fallen victim to a minor dispute or emotional breakdown. One woman reported feeling so 'irrationally' upset that the dishwasher had failed to properly clean a wine glass that she, quite uncharacteristically, threw the glass against a nearby wall; this required not just a replacement glass, but a re-plastering job too. So, whether its flying saucers, harsh words or just a whole load of tears, it would be remarkable if you and your partner got through an entire pregnancy without a similar story to tell. Pregnancy is a tense - sometimes very stressful - time with nature's hormones kicking your partner pretty hard now and again. No matter what happens, try to keep your cool. It will pass.

The first antenatal appointment is an exciting time for most couples as it all starts to feel more real, but I've been disappointed by the number of dads who have said that they were made to feel like a spare part. Of course, there'll be a moment when they ask you to leave the room and we all know that you're not, hopefully, going to be pushing anything out of your pelvis when the big day finally comes, but chances are you are still the best supporter, advocate and ultimately co-parent your partner has. Most modern, open-minded healthcare professionals appreciate this; in fact, we now know that dads also undergo physical and hormonal changes during pregnancy, which lead to an increased level of the hormone oxytocin and even changes in the part of the brain responsible for nurturing and problem solving. So, don't settle for being seated in the corner like a naughty schoolboy; if you want to be involved, make that happen. Luckily, most healthcare professionals involved in bringing babies into the world love all things childbirth-related, so a few sensible and caring questions from you should seal your place at the pregnancy discussion table.

I found the early days of pregnancy strange. It was a bit like making a massive decision to quit your job, telling your boss, but then having to serve out your three-month notice period. I'd taken the huge decision to try for a baby. We'd been successful and all the paperwork was being completed, but slightly anti-climactically, for me nothing really changed for the first few months - flying crockery aside. Underlying it all was a niggling worry in the back of my mind that something might, quite conceivably, go wrong. I've given the sad news of miscarriage to many couples, but could do nothing about my own baby except keep everything crossed in the hope that things would continue smoothly over the painstakingly slow weeks that followed.

What Women Want

DO discuss who, if anyone, you're going to tell about the pregnancy during the first trimester.

DON'T expect your partner to stay up late or have loads of energy. The first trimester is exhausting.

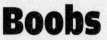

Boobs

The good, the bad and the... changes of pregnancy

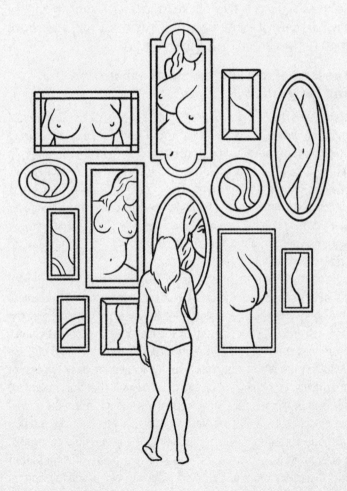

FROM THE DOCTOR

Everything is now changing, developing and growing – both inside and out. The first trimester is the phase of pregnancy where the greatest changes occur in the shortest period of time, so being prepared to be especially supportive of your partner throughout these first few months is vital. The change from fertile woman to pregnant mother takes its toll on the body both mentally, but you already know that, and physically. While the mental changes are often the most discussed by dads, thanks to those seemingly pointless arguments they can generate, women usually find the physical burden the greatest and this in turn may have a significant impact on their mental health too.

The land of morning sickness, exhaustion and indigestion

Sometimes the first sign of pregnancy is the nausea or vomiting of 'morning sickness'. Not really a brilliantly named feature of pregnancy, because although it often occurs in the morning, in reality it can occur at any time of day and for many women this beast is, sadly, not confined to a few queasy hours as the sun starts to rise. If you imagine that feeling of nausea caused by a hangover from a particularly heavy night suddenly hitting you without warning on an almost daily basis, you'll go some way to understanding how unpleasant it can be.

Nobody knows for sure what causes morning sickness, though our old friends the hormones hCG and oestrogen are often blamed. One theory is that it's due to relaxation of the muscles in the stomach and intestine, caused by the elevated levels of pregnancy hormones that lead to all the misery, but the jury's still out. It's fiendishly common and has usually kicked in by 9 weeks of pregnancy, if not earlier, but the good news is that, for around 90 per cent of women, this unwelcome nemesis has normally moved on by week 16 if not earlier, although a few unlucky women continue to suffer beyond this point. It's impossible to predict who's going to get the worst cases of the queasy nastiness, but your partner's more at risk if she's having her first baby, suffers with travel or motion sickness, has migraines, is obese or has a family history of women with bad morning sickness. It's also more common in women carrying twins or multiple pregnancies, which may give some support to the high hormone level argument.

Fortunately for most women, the nausea and vomiting cause no harm at all to the baby on board, but the bad news is that there's no treatment for it other than time. For most it can be added to the list of pregnancy unpleasantries and it's soon forgotten once the first trimester moves aside. There are some tips that can definitely help relieve the symptoms though, such as eating small, regular meals and avoiding any foods or smells that make them heave or want to run to the nearest bathroom to empty the contents of their newly filled stomach. Having a small snack on waking can really make a difference – leave a pack of plain crackers on the bedside table for her to devour as soon as she's awake in the morning. Women often report that symptoms are much worse if they don't eat until later in the day, so getting something plain and simple in early doors can really make a difference. Others find ginger helpful, whether it's eating a biscuit, crushing it into a juice or even sniffing a freshly cut piece of ginger root. Again, the science here is limited at best, but when needs must, most things have got to be worth a try – there's certainly no harm in giving it a go. Some women swear by acupuncture, but others never find anything that helps. If none of the traditional remedies are really cutting it, then get your partner along to see her doctor, who can prescribe anti-sickness medication, safe for pregnancy, that will hopefully make everything much more bearable. Let's not forget the lucky ones, though, who have no morning sickness at all – this is also completely normal and shouldn't lead to stress about how well the pregnancy's progressing – just count your lucky stars.

A few women suffer very severe symptoms in a condition known as hyperemesis gravidarum, a Greek–Latin hybrid meaning 'excessive vomiting of the pregnant', which is exactly what it says on the tin. Severe vomiting prevents these women from keeping down any food or drink, which can lead to dehydration and signs of starvation. When the body doesn't have enough food to break down and convert into energy, it starts to break down body fat and this leads to the production of ketones in the urine, which can be detected using urine test strips. If your partner is suffering from severe vomiting, she should be assessed by a healthcare professional to see whether she is developing signs of hyperemesis gravidarum. If she is, she may need to be admitted to hospital for re-hydration with intravenous fluids and some super-strength anti-sickness medications.

Feeling a bit queasy yourself Dad? Well, you're not alone. A proportion of male partners report feeling pregnancy-associated symptoms too. Known as Couvade Syndrome, this is a poorly understood phenomenon, but certainly one that's well recognized, with men describing symptoms from nausea to mood swings and bloating. Experts argue over the reasons behind it and many feel it's a result of the psychological changes dads-to-be are undergoing. If you find yourself feeling a bit out of sorts, perhaps a 'sympathetic' pregnancy is the cause?

Whether or not the nausea is kicking in, indigestion and acid reflux are very likely to feature on the complaints list as pregnancy gets underway. Relaxation of the sphincter muscle that stops acid rising up out of the stomach into the food pipe (gullet, or oesophagus) can cause horrible heartburn, so get in early with antacids and encourage your partner to avoid spicy or acidic foods that might trigger symptoms. Some antacids work by forming a protective layer over the top of the sea of stomach acid, preventing it from irritating the walls of the oesophagus above. If these aren't enough to control the burping and burning, try a medication that reduces the production of stomach acid. You can buy them over the counter at a pharmacy.

Physical changes start earlier than you think

Moving upwards and sideways from the stomach and heartburn leads us neatly to the boobs. Breast changes happen earlier than you, or your partner, might have expected in pregnancy as the hormones ready the intricate mountains of ducts and glands to provide a buffet of dreams once the baby arrives. For new mums and dads, this is probably the first time you've really considered the genuine practical benefits of breasts. Some will love the enlarging nipples, the darkening skin around them and ever-increasing size of the boobs themselves. However, others may be a bit unnerved by the occasional discharge or milky leak that comes a-flowing as the milk machine prepares for action. Your excitement at the sudden increase in cup size – if that's your thing – may be met with unfortunate disapproval by your partner though. Breasts are often very tender during the first trimester and you may find the only real boob action you're getting is accompanying your partner as the search for a bigger more supportive bra begins. Handle with care.

Across the chest wall another change that you may both have noticed is the arrival of a meshwork of thin blue lines, commoner in fair-skinned or thin women. These veins, which look like a spider has gone into overdrive, spinning a veiny web over your partner's chest, are completely normal. During pregnancy blood volume (and flow) increases to provide the body with all the nutrients required for baby carrying. This increase around the breasts leads to the presence of these mysterious thin blue lines and they may appear elsewhere on the body too. These so-called 'spider veins', thin, wispy, blue-purple veins may pop up on the legs or abdomen. They're not the prettiest of additions, but mainly unavoidable.

The increased blood volume, combined with the pressure of an ever-growing uterus pushing on the veins carrying blood from the legs back to the heart, reduces their formerly uninterrupted free-flow, which can lead to varicose veins. These raised and sometimes unsightly leg veins are one of the other aesthetic hazards of pregnancy. More common in those who spend a lot of their day standing – chefs, surgeons and policewomen beware – they can be hard to avoid. If your partner exercises regularly to promote blood flow and puts her feet up when sitting or lying down that will help the return of blood from the legs and keep the risk of varicose veins to a minimum. Most varicose veins will settle once pregnancy is over, but for those that persist, surgical removal is an option and can give excellent results – though it's not advisable until several months after baby is born.

While we're checking out your partner's legs, remember that pregnancy brings with it the increased risk of blood clots in the legs – what's known as a deep vein thrombosis, or DVT. The hormonal changes lead to 'stickier' blood that is more likely to clot, so be on the lookout for a swollen, painful or red calf or thigh that may be the first sign of an underlying blood clot. Reduced mobility, such as on long car journeys or long-haul flights as well as dehydration, increase the risk. If you're jetting off across the world with your partner or sitting still for hours on end, encourage regular breaks with time to walk around and embrace all those exercises airlines now include in their inflight magazines. The rather embarrassing, tip-toe stand-ups or the ankle-swirling dance may make you both look a bit un-travel chic, but they could prevent dangerous clots forming.

Down below things are changing too. And yes, by down below I do mean the vagina. Discharge often increases significantly during pregnancy and strangely enough, while morning sickness and indigestion get all the attention, few women discuss the massive change in vaginal secretion they've noticed in pregnancy so it often catches them and their partners by surprise. Sometimes it's so severe that a pad is required. You may also notice a change in the smell of vaginal discharge, which, combined with a leaky boob, can lead to a whole host of new nasal scent discoveries in the bedroom. All of these are likely to revert to normal after birth, and it's just the start of the bodily fluids you're going to become accustomed to over the months ahead. So, support your partner – just simply understanding that it's normal, not disgusting, will make a massive difference.

What's happening to the baby?

It's the mega-changes deep inside the uterus that would really blow your mind – if only you could see them. Since the sperm–egg combo first started to develop into an embryo, then implanted into the wall of the uterus, cells have been dividing at break-neck speed. You don't need to become an embryologist, but a basic understanding of what's happening might help. In the early weeks the developing embryo forms into three layers: the outer layer (ectoderm), middle layer (mesoderm) and the inner layer (endoderm). The outer layer goes on to form the 'neural tube' from which the brain, spinal cord and nerves all develop – it's this layer that is helped along its way by those trusty folic acid supplements your partner's struggling to remember to take each day. From the middle layer arise the bones and the muscles – including that most important muscle of all, the heart. The inner layer forms the squidgy insides of humans like the lungs, bowel and the urinary tract. A miracle of engineering is now occurring as you watch blissfully unaware from the next-door pillow.

By the fifth week small 'buds' appear that will eventually develop into arms and legs. At the same time, the heart begins to divide into chambers, then somewhere around the six-week mark, it begins to start beating. Facial features are also starting to emerge – dark spots appear at the site where openings for eyes, mouth and nostrils will soon start to form – but it's not going to be possible to tell who that baby looks like quite yet. So, for those tempted by the idea of an early scan, bear in mind that there will be very little to see before 6–8 weeks and it's not until then that you're likely to be able to see that all-important beat of a tiny, tiny heart.

FROM THE DAD

As a hater of nausea, the thought of morning sickness as a daily hangover-sensation, lasting months, fills me with horror. It's such a weird and unpleasant way for a woman to begin her pregnancy journey, but it's the first diagnosis that pops into my head when a woman of childbearing age comes into clinic complaining of feeling nauseous. It's always a little embarrassing for a doctor to blame last night's curry when it turns out to be a baby not the Balti causing the symptoms. My wife felt pretty sick for the first 12 weeks, but luckily only actually vomited on a few special occasions. About 10 weeks into the pregnancy, we went to a wedding with a large group of close friends. Trying to keep the pregnancy under wraps suddenly became more difficult than just silently necking my wife's champagne when the vomit made an appearance. To make matters worse, she was meant to be singing during the wedding service. 'No, I'm not hungover. No, I'm not sick with nerves,' she told them. 'So, you must be... suffering very bad food poisoning', came the response. Obviously.

Our bedroom soon become littered with left-over packets of dried biscuits or half-eaten snacks gobbled down at bizarre hours of the night and began to look as if a group of out-of-control kids had rented it for a sleepover complete with midnight feasts. But simply eating a little food immediately upon waking really did the trick and helped settle the nausea almost instantly. Other dads' tales of their partner vomiting at least daily are all too common, but sadly many women report a lack of sympathy from their employers. Most weeks on duty in the emergency department involved admitting at least one woman with hyperemesis gravidarum. One dad-to-be accompanying his partner confessed that he hadn't been to the department since he'd been hospitalized with similar symptoms after a particularly big night out and was devastated to hear that his partner had become so unwell through absolutely no fault of her own. Luckily, thanks to anti-sickness medications and the wonders of intravenous fluids, mums can normally be turned around pretty quickly, so if vomiting appears out of control, be sure to get some help for your partner.

Look carefully around your office and you may be able to spot a covertly pregnant woman by the tell-tale sign of a massive bottle of antacid medication sitting on her desk. Reflux or indigestion is often worsened by specific foods, particularly those with more acidic contents. Red peppers were one nemesis that regularly sent a colleague of mine into a corner to gulp on her antacid brand of choice. You can only hope that the pregnancy cravings and indigestion triggers don't coincide. I'd imagined that my wife would be ramping up her normal love of the odd chocolate bar or be craving some expensive luxury caviar that she'd never even tried before, but for her the cravings didn't feature as highly as dislikes and even disgusts. For three months the woman I love, but who certainly loves chocolate more than me, could not go near the stuff. One weekend, in a slightly lazy moment of friend-entertaining, with a heavily pregnant vegetarian wife also to cater for, I bought a ready-roasted chicken for the few people we had coming over. Imagine the shock when I entered the kitchen to find my wife, who had not eaten meat for more than four years ripping the chicken meat off the bone with her bare hands and shoving it into her mouth like a hungry lioness who'd successfully annihilated her prey. Not a sliver of meat has been eaten since, but don't let anybody tell you these pregnancy cravings aren't powerful when they strike.

I was shocked by how early on in pregnancy the physical changes started to kick in. Boobs were definitely the first to balloon and it wasn't as good as you might imagine. In fact, they were so sensitive that for several weeks we were unable to hug without me being reprimanded for coming into vague contact with the developing ducts of milky goodness. Instead, like a personal shopper on his first day in the lingerie department, I stood lovingly by as the benefits of push-up versus balconette bras were debated. But rewards were reaped. A comfortable, supportive, (definitely not underwired) new bra made the world of difference - with sports bras coming out top. This could be an ideal early pregnancy gift if you're a little more size-savvy than me. Pleasingly, the breast tenderness did settle down as the weeks went by and it wasn't until the milk started coming in after birth that we found ourselves back - this time online - at the virtual lingerie department.

What Women Want

DO expect mood swings and be tolerant when they occur.

DO have a constant supply of biscuits available to help fight off the morning sickness.

DON'T try to squeeze your partner's blossoming, but hugely delicate and painful breasts. It really hurts!

DON'T tell you partner that she is looking fatter or that her body is ballooning.

5

Heart

Pulses racing for the first scan

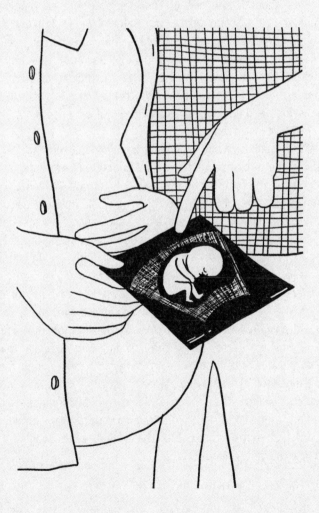

FROM THE DOCTOR

Some couples just simply cannot wait to get that first glimpse of their baby, so much so that they come to ask me whether they should have an 'early' scan, before the standard dating scan that's offered at around 12 weeks. If your partner's had any complications, like bleeding or abdominal pain, so far in her pregnancy, you may well have had a peek at your ever-growing piece of handiwork already. Some clinics will offer a scan before 12 weeks, but if you're thinking about it you should consider a couple of important reminders. First, scanning too early, before 6 weeks, is likely to be disappointing as you may not see a foetal heartbeat even if everything is going swimmingly inside. Secondly, the risk of miscarriage significantly reduces after 12 weeks' gestation, so scanning before this may lead to an increased emotional burden if things don't end up going as expected. But if patience is not your strong point – then scan away.

If the pregnancy has been progressing as normal and you've resisted the temptation to check out your future offspring at an early stage, the first meeting you're likely to have – at least via a computer screen – is at the so-called 12-week 'dating scan'. For those guys saving up their leave allowance for antenatal appointments, this should definitely be the one at the top of the 'not to be missed' list. A sonographer – that's an ultrasound specialist – or a doctor will use an ultrasound probe to scan your partner's uterus and, all being well, show you your baby for the very first time. This scan is normally performed over the tummy, not with a vaginal probe, involves lots of jelly and some pretty firm pushing by the person doing the scanning and normally takes 15–30 minutes to complete. It's not always the most comfortable experience for mum. Having plenty of water to drink, and a full bladder, can help make things easier to see, but imagine really needing a pee and somebody pushing on your tummy – not ideal. So, don't let your partner overdo the drinking or the whole thing can become quite uncomfortable.

What happens at the dating scan?

It won't be long before you can see a black-and-white image of your baby up on the screen for the very first time. There's no evidence to suggest that ultrasound scanning causes any damage to your baby, and rest assured, having a scan doesn't lead to any recognized complications or increase the risk of miscarriage either. It does take patience though. Sometimes it takes a few minutes to get things in focus, so no panicking if you can't quite see that image you've become so used to seeing all over social media straight away. After what may seem like an eternity to you, the sonographer will zoom in on the heart and hopefully you'll be able to hear baby's heartbeat for the first time. Sounding like something somewhere between a pumping heart and alien communication, this tiny vital organ should be beating at around 160 beats per minute. Even if your nerves and excitement are now sky high, this is still likely to be much faster than your own heart rate; a child's heart rate slows to a normal adult rate from the age of about twelve.

A few very important checks are carried out during this scan. The length of your baby is measured from the head to the buttocks, known as the crown-to-rump length, or CRL. This gives a more accurate gestational age and enables the sonographer to update the estimated delivery date from the period-based calculation you spent all that time doing a few weeks back. They'll then move on to have a brief look at the baby's limbs and organs, the skull and brain, the arms and legs as well as organs such as the stomach, bowel and bladder.

One seemingly random, but very important measurement is the thickness of the back of the baby's neck, what is known as 'nuchal thickness'. Increased fluid in this normally occurring fold at the back of the neck can suggest an increased risk of genetic disorders, such as Down's syndrome. More on genetic screening in Chapter 6, but this measurement when combined with a blood test can give a risk estimate of various genetic disorders.

As well as baby, the sonographer will also look at the position of the placenta within the uterus. Most of the time the placenta attaches to the side of the uterus, away from the exit, or cervix, that baby will come through during vaginal delivery. In some pregnancies the placenta is 'low lying' and very close to the exit, so much so that it may get in the way during delivery – known as placenta praevia. Luckily, as the uterus grows, the placenta is often drawn upwards and out of the way, but your healthcare team will keep a closer eye if they think there's a risk of it blocking the exit route.

One key piece of information you can't find out at this scan is the sex of your baby. Even if you have decided you want to know, it's too early in the growth process to give information about gender now. Of course, the sex of your baby was determined way back at conception by the sex chromosomes it's inherited from you, but for now, the boy-girl mystery continues, so don't expect a big reveal. A potential surprise that may not have crossed your mind is that today could be the day you find out you're going to father twins or even triplets. Pregnancies with multiple foetuses require much closer monitoring and this will be taken care of by your healthcare team, but it's worth bearing in mind that this scan might reveal that there's more than one baby lurking in there.

With the measurements all done and the new estimated delivery date (EDD) firmly etched on your mind, it's now time for that all-important photo. If you'd like a copy of the scan pictures most units are happy to provide these for you, but some will charge for the privilege, so be sure to take along some loose change as they often won't accept payment by card.

Seeing your baby on the screen for the very first time can lead to a whole host of different emotions in both you and your partner. Relief, delight, nervous anxiety or simply the sudden realization that this is really happening. In just a few months, a baby is coming your way. Tears are very common and for many the sheer relief of seeing that all is well and hearing the heartbeat for the first time can be quite overwhelming, so have some tissues ready. Occasionally an abnormality is noticed during the scan and your partner may be referred to a foetal medicine specialist for further testing or scanning.

Very sadly, for some parents, the 12-week scan brings bad news when the baby's heart is found not to be beating. At this stage of pregnancy it can occur without any warning signs and is known as 'silent miscarriage'. Such sad news will inevitably come as a considerable shock and can be particularly difficult to take on board if there have been no concerns up until this point. Allow yourselves time to discuss the situation with your team as there will be some difficult decisions ahead as to how best to manage the miscarriage. Some mothers choose to wait and let nature take its course with careful supervision while others are advised or prefer to use medications or surgical miscarriage management.

Letting the secret out

All being well, you're now armed with your black-and-white ultrasound printout and desperate to reveal to the world the secret you've been keeping for the last few months. Many couples wait until the dating scan before announcing their pregnancy because the reassurance of a normal scan combined with the approaching start of the second trimester means that the risk of miscarriage is now significantly reduced. So, whether you're planning social media announcements, cards for your nearest and dearest or even a comedy announcement video, now's the time to get creative. It's always worth bearing in mind that friends around you may be struggling to conceive or suffering as a result of recent miscarriages. Don't feel that this is a reason not to celebrate your happy news but remain mindful of the fact that some couples may be finding life a bit tougher.

As well as the relief of being about to share the news, the end of the first trimester and the start of the second often brings with it an overall feeling of improvement for your partner. Morning sickness symptoms will usually begin to settle and those radical variations in mood will also reduce. Many women describe the second trimester as the best phase of pregnancy with the unpleasant symptoms of the early weeks behind them and the full physical strain of carrying an increasingly large human in your belly yet to really strike.

New symptoms kick in

While many symptoms are settling, inevitably they'll be replaced by some new ones. The breasts are still on the rise and hormones are flying around the bloodstream. The bowels and bladder really start to get involved too now. Many women suffer with constipation during pregnancy. The hormone progesterone relaxes the bowel, so the business doesn't pass through as quickly as normal and that, combined with the increasing pressure in the pelvic area from the heavily laden uterus, means things can start to get bunged up. High-fibre foods are helpful, like whole-grain cereals and brown rice as well as plenty of fruit and vegetables. Keeping well hydrated is vital to keep the bowels moving, aiming for at least 2 litres of fluid daily. Regular exercise will also help to keep the motions flowing.

Straining to open her bowels will increase your partner's risk of developing haemorrhoids, small blood vessels, normally present around the entrance to the bum (anus), that can become enlarged in pregnancy. Haemorrhoids can be itchy, sometimes painful and can bleed, leading to fresh red blood being found on toilet tissue after wiping or in the toilet bowl itself. Check first that the blood is definitely from the bum and not the vagina, and then relax a little. Haemorrhoids are very common and can be easily treated with over-the-counter creams that are safe to use in pregnancy. Applying them is a bit fiddly and gross, but symptoms should be under control in no time. If there's bleeding that won't settle or the haemorrhoids become very painful, then encourage your partner to have them checked by a healthcare professional.

Partner peeing all the time? No surprises there. Those trusty pregnancy hormones increase the blood volume and also increase the blood flow to the kidneys. As the kidneys do their vital filtering role, large volumes of urine are produced, and we all know what that means – a desperate need for a wee just at the most inconvenient moment as well as nights spent running back and forth to the bathroom. A similar feeling to having had a few pints of beer, made worse by the pressure of a growing uterus and baby pushing on the bladder.

The ever-increasing weight carried in your partner's pelvis –

the part of the body carrying the uterus, bladder and bowels – can lead to weakness in the muscles supporting the pelvic floor. If you're not quite sure which muscles these are, try this little experiment. Next time you're having a wee, stop suddenly. That's them. The very muscles you squeeze to stop the flow of urine are those of the pelvic floor. They will be weakened by the pressure of pregnancy and, in a few months' time, by the passage of a baby through the birth canal. Now is a perfect time to encourage your partner to start some pelvic-floor exercises. Regularly exercising these muscles, like any other muscles, increases their strength and reduces the risk of incontinence later. Regular squeezing of the muscles, using that 'stop the pee' technique, is all it takes and there are loads of different apps available to remind her when to squeeze throughout the day. In fact, why not join in yourself. Pelvic-floor exercises can reduce premature ejaculation in men – everybody's winning now.

Now that you're both exercising your pelvic floors, your partner might be wondering what other exercise it's appropriate to do during pregnancy. Keeping fit and healthy is likely to both help with labour and make it easier for your partner to get back in shape after giving birth. Sensible activities are not dangerous for your baby so your partner should continue any that she used to take before becoming pregnant. She may become tired more quickly and should listen to her body, avoid doing anything overly strenuous and aim to still be able to hold a conversation while exercising. If your partner wasn't active prior to pregnancy she shouldn't suddenly start vigorous exercise but start something gentle – even just walking to the shops will make a difference. Swimming, pregnancy yoga and Pilates are all excellent while the bump continues to grow, as they help to strengthen core muscles and maintain general fitness. Sports that may cause harm to the unborn baby should obviously be avoided, especially those where there's a risk of the baby being hit, such as rugby, kickboxing or martial arts. Your partner should not SCUBA dive because of the risk of decompression sickness in your unborn child and should seek advice if travelling to high altitudes. Remember that little black-and-white ball of baby human you saw on the scan – help your partner to guard them well. It won't be long before baby's out and she's back to the base jumping, rugby tackling, karate-fuelled life of days gone by – childcare dependent obviously.

FROM THE DAD

As a couple, it's fair to say we are both pretty impatient. I couldn't wait to see what was going on inside and to get that first glimpse of our baby. Pregnancy seemed to have coincided with a run of really close friends getting married and to avoid too many suspicious questions, as well as any fear of stealing limelight on somebody else's big day, we'd decided to let a few of our nearest and dearest in on the secret early, before the scheduled 12-week dating scan. So, before giving any news to anybody we arranged a scan. A local private clinic was offering a discount on 'early pregnancy' scans, so one evening after work at around 8 weeks, off we set, hoping to see signs of life in the uterus for the very first time. I was extremely cautious. I don't know if this came from hours spent in early pregnancy assessment units seeing couples receive the sad news of miscarriage – in which case I can just blame being a doctor for my anxiety – or whether I would have felt like this anyway. I had messaged my wife earlier that day warning her that we 'might receive sad news tonight'. What a kill-joy!

The nervous wait in the clinic's reception soon turned into what felt like the set of a sit-com. Women were coming out from scans squealing with delight, grandmothers-to-be were debating whether or not £5 was a bargain for a DVD of their future grandchild and a down-trodden dad was looking furious about the £25 he'd just parted with for a teddy bear that played, on demand, the sound of his child's foetal heartbeat. My intense fear of the sonographer saying that they couldn't find a heartbeat actually took away from my enjoyment of the experience. When the flashing, beating, whooshing heartbeat quickly appeared on the screen, rather than sheer delight, I just felt a massive sense of relief. I'd also got very excited about the possibility of discovering we were having twins, but on this occasion the sonographer found just one new addition growing safely within. Most dads I've spoken to report some anxiety ahead of the first scan, but I think, like my wife, I'm going to blame my medical training for my unnecessarily pessimistic outlook. Try to master the balance of anxiety and that joyous first peek better than I did if you possibly can.

By the time the scheduled 12-week dating scan came around I was much more relaxed. Seeing what you, as a couple, have created - quite literally in black and white - on the screen in front of you is nothing short of miraculous. While my wife had been battling for months with the first trimester of pregnancy, vomiting, feeling exhausted and collating a wardrobe of elastic-waisted jeans, it wasn't until I sat staring at my future child on the screen before me that the reality of what lay ahead truly hit me. I suddenly lost all interest in the measurements or science that normally would have fascinated me. My mind was elsewhere - thinking about nappies, finances and sleep deprivation. I wondered: 'Would they get married?', 'Who would they look like?', 'What if they got bullied at school?', 'What would be their first word?'. It was in that moment that I truly transitioned from doctor to dad-to-be.

What Women Want

DO talk through the tests that your partner is going to undergo and discuss any anxieties you both have about them.

DON'T rush to spread the news on social media - or anywhere else - before your partner is ready. Follow her lead.

6

Genes

The science of screening

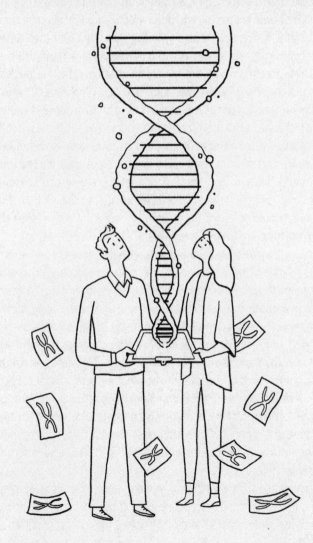

FROM THE DOCTOR

Every cell in our body, except for a man's sperm and a woman's eggs, contains our specific DNA packaged into 23 pairs of genetic bundles, known as chromosomes – 46 in total. Each sperm and egg contain a 'single string' or just 23 single chromosomes. At conception, 23 of mum's chromosomes meet 23 of dad's chromosomes and this newly combined ball of DNA then becomes the half-mum, half-dad foetus we've been talking about all this time. Historically, it was the women who got into trouble if they didn't produce the male offspring required as heirs – think Henry VIII and his falsely accused wives. We know now that one of these pairs of chromosomes are what we call 'sex chromosomes', which determine the gender of the baby. If an X chromosome is paired with a Y chromosome then you'll have yourself a male foetus, while two X's gives you a female. As it's the Y chromosome that makes a baby male and women don't carry this chromosome, it's the man who has a 50 per cent chance of making his offspring male. Personally, even if I had been alive and in possession of this knowledge during Henry VII's reign, I'd rather not have been the one to tell him – he sounds pretty scary.

So, you're probably thinking, how else do these chromosomes fit into our tale of baby-making? It's becoming increasingly common for couples to wait until later in life to have children and many are concerned about the risks that advancing age might bring during pregnancy. The good news is that, although there are risks associated with women over the age of 35 having children, they are still relatively small and usually far outweighed by the huge benefits of parenthood, which is important to remember as we look at them in more detail. If you're reading thinking, my partner's not over 35 and nor am I, don't flick to the next chapter quite yet. Whatever your partner's age, she'll be offered screening tests for common genetic disorders, so a basic understanding of what you're letting yourselves in for is vital.

Women are born with their lifetime's supply of eggs already on board, but their reserves decline with time, and run out at the menopause. Women of 35 and older have a higher risk of suffering with fertility issues and a greater risk of miscarriage. Us men on the other hand start to produce sperm later on and continue to do so on a daily basis well into old age. As women age they're also more likely to release more than one egg each month and therefore they have a higher chance of conceiving twins or triplets.

Now back to our friend the chromosome. As women age there is a greater risk of chromosomal damage that may result in a baby with a genetic (inherited) disorder. There are thousands of different recognized – and many thousands of as-yet unrecognized – genetic disorders, but we'll stick to the big names here. Also, if you know that you, or members of your family, carry or are at risk of a particular disorder, be sure to discuss this with your healthcare team at the earliest opportunity.

One common genetic error happens when an uninvited third chromosome joins one of the normal 23 pairs – a phenomenon known as trisomy. Down's syndrome is caused by three copies of chromosome 21; three copies of chromosome 18 results in Edward's syndrome and Patau syndrome occurs if there are three copies of chromosome 13. The chances of your child having Down's syndrome increase with maternal age. A mum in her 20s has around a one in 1,500 chance of having an affected child, in her 30s it's one in 800, by the age of 35 the risk increases to one in 270 and by age 40 to one in 100. It used to be thought that only the mother's age mattered, but more recent studies suggest that increasing paternal age also has an impact. When getting your head around all this, don't forget that any mother, at any age, could have a child with a genetic disorder such as Down's Syndrome. All parents strive for a 'healthy child', so screening tests have been put in place to give you and your partner more information about your child's specific risks.

It's possible to screen for risks

Screening can assess the risk of a baby having a genetic condition. One such test, known as the 'combined test', assesses for the risk of Down's, Edward's and Patau syndromes and must be carried out before 14 weeks of pregnancy. First, the nuchal translucency (the thickness of the fold at the back of the baby's neck, page 49) –

is measured by ultrasound at the dating scan. Next up is a blood test for mum to measure the levels of two substances: human chorionic gonadotrophin (hCG) – of the pregnancy test fame – and the pregnancy-associated plasma protein A, or PAPP-A. The results are then interpreted alongside, or 'combined' with, maternal age and medical history to give a theoretical risk of the child being born with one of these conditions.

If your partner didn't manage to have the combined test before she was 14 weeks pregnant, she can have a 'quadruple test' up to 20 weeks. This is a simple blood test that measures the levels of two hormones – hCG and oestriol – and two proteins – alpha fetoprotein (AFP) and inhibin A – which, when interpreted in the context of age and medical history, can also be used to calculate baby's risk profile. This test is less reliable than the combined test.

The latest development in antenatal screening, known as Non-invasive Prenatal Testing, or NIPT, was previously only available privately. It's been established that small fragments of foetal DNA from the placenta travel in the mother's blood stream and a simple maternal blood test can be used to screen the DNA for chromo-somal abnormalities, like Down's syndrome, in her baby. This test is highly accurate and picks up around 99 per cent of those who are later confirmed to have the condition. NIPT can be carried out any time from 10 weeks' gestation and as an added bonus, if you and your partner wish, it can also tell you the sex of your baby months before it can be seen on an ultrasound scan.

The world of diagnostic tests

Whichever screening tests your healthcare team are offering, they don't give a diagnosis; they're simply tools that indicate the likelihood, or not, of your unborn child having a genetic disorder. The benefit of the screening tests is that they don't harm the baby or increase the risk of miscarraige. As with any test, they can sometimes be incorrect, either giving false reassurance that everything's fine or raising concern about a baby who turns out to be completely healthy. For example, about one in 300 NIPTs give a false positive – suggesting that a baby has Down's when in fact it doesn't.

If your partner's screening tests show an increased risk of an underlying disorder, particularly if that risk is greater than one in 150, your healthcare team will offer a diagnostic test. These are also offered to mums who've had previous pregnancies with chromosomal abnormalities, those with a family history of genetic disorders like cystic fibrosis, sickle-cell disease or thalassaemia, or women who have had an abnormal finding on an ultrasound scan. Remember, too, that your partner doesn't have to undergo these diagnostic tests, and it's important for you both to weigh up the pros and cons of testing and not testing very carefully by discussing it with her team. There are two invasive tests offered – amniocentesis and chorionic villus sampling. Both can provide a definitive diagnosis, but they aren't without their risks.

Amniotic fluid is the watery liquid within the amniotic sac that surrounds baby in the uterus and it contains foetal cells from the baby. Amniocentesis is a procedure where, under the guidance of ultrasound, a small sample of this fluid is removed using a needle passed through the abdominal wall and into the uterus. It's normally done between weeks 15 and 20 of pregnancy. The doctor numbs the skin using a local anaesthetic. Most mums don't find it painful, just a bit uncomfortable. Some say they feel a period-like cramping pain during the procedure.

Chorionic villus sampling, or CVS, is a similar procedure, but with this test the sample is taken from the cells of the placenta itself. This time, depending on where the placenta is sitting, the needle can either be passed through the abdominal wall or through the neck of the uterus, or cervix, and yes, a local anaesthetic is always given. CVS can be performed at an earlier stage of pregnancy, usually between 11 and 14 weeks.

Both tests carry a small, but not insignificant, risk of miscarriage, with rates of 0.5 to 1 per cent being quoted; the risk following CVS is slightly higher than for amniocentesis. There's also a small risk of bleeding and infection after both procedures, and rhesus-negative mums (see Chapter 3) will require an Anti-D injection to cover any possible exposure to foetal blood.

Once the samples have been taken, they're sent away for analysis, with rapid test results being available within about 3 days, while more complex genetic tests take up to two weeks to come back. In most instances, the test will give a clear 'yes' or 'no' answer, potentially leaving you both with some difficult decisions to discuss and make. The majority of conditions being tested for don't, at present, have a cure, so it's important to weigh up your options carefully. Some parents choose to proceed with the pregnancy, finding out as much about the condition as possible to let them prepare for baby's arrival. Others may decide not to continue with the pregnancy and discuss the options for termination (abortion) with their healthcare team.

It would be wrong for me to give specific advice about what to do in these situations. Each condition is unique with its own list of potential complications; some, all or none of which may affect your child. The decision to continue with a pregnancy needs to be carefully considered and all of your individual circumstances, beliefs and opinions need to be taken into consideration. The ultimate decision rests with the mother carrying the baby, but of course, a jointly discussed and mutually agreed outcome will make coping with whichever path you ultimately choose as a couple far easier to follow. Accurate information is going to be crucial here, so be sure to access all of the specialists and resources available to you. Some couples find it helpful to discuss their thoughts on genetic disorders and termination of pregnancy prior to undertaking screening tests, as it's sometimes easier to have a rational discussion outside the heated pressure of emotionally fuelled decision-making. So, it's perhaps a topic of conversation for one of those pregnancy-friendly dinners you've cooked up for your partner in the early weeks.

FROM THE DAD

Six weeks after I was born my parents were told I had the genetic condition albinism. This is a defect in the gene that makes the pigment melanin - which gives skin and hair its colour. Melanin also helps the retina at the back of the eye to develop, so people with albinism also have varying degrees of visual impairment. So, my parents had produced a whiter than white baby whose eyes didn't work very well. At the time, the doctors generally painted a pretty grim picture, telling my parents that I would never be able to go to a normal school and would struggle to lead a normal life. Luckily, thanks to a lot of support from family and friends, a large amount of determination and some even larger font textbooks, none of these warnings became a reality - well, except for the eyesight, which is pretty poor. Neither of my parents, nor anybody else in my family, has albinism, but both of them carried a copy of the faulty gene and passed it to me - resulting, for better or worse, in the person I am today.

I've always worried about passing albinism on to my child, knowing that whatever I did and however my cells divided, all of my sperm would carry a copy of the faulty gene. Not making babies with another person with albinism was one way of reducing the chance of passing this on. But how did I know that my wife didn't also carry a copy of the gene? Well I didn't. But when we started thinking about baby-making, I had a chat with a geneticist who advised me that if we weren't related and there wasn't any history of albinism in my wife's family, the chances of her being a carrier were very low - but not non-existent. So, as long as my gene didn't meet another albinism gene, any child of mine would escape the genetic roulette unscathed.

I'm not sure many couples are truly able to consider the impact of having a child with a genetic disorder, whether that's Down's syndrome, albinism, cystic fibrosis or any other, before the baby arrives. Like imagining how it will feel to finally become a dad, it's one of those concepts you never fully grasp until you're living the reality on a daily basis - no matter how informative the books you read might be. After a lengthy discussion, my wife and I decided three things. First, we wanted to have a child, secondly, we wanted that to be with each other and, thirdly, despite the significant disability afforded to me by albinism I have had a fulfilling, high-achieving life so far and if anyone could support a person with albinism, we could. I still didn't love the prospect though.

I was worried, mainly, for my wife. She'd always imagined herself being a mum one day, but she hadn't even contemplated finding a husband with faulty genes - now she had to. Would it change our relationship? Would she feel that I was to blame? But when we delved further, we decided that on many levels none of our genes were perfect. Luckily, we didn't know of any life-limiting genetic disorders that we carried but, of course, it may have been faulty genes that we were blissfully unaware of that could cause our offspring their biggest problems.

Just as we were at the height of genetic discussions, I met a very anxious mum who'd brought her child into my clinic with a fever. There was nothing seriously wrong, but she explained to me that ever since her pregnancy she had been extremely concerned about her child's health. It turned out that this all stemmed from the NIPT testing she had undergone during her early pregnancy. As low-risk parents they'd expected a normal result, but the test had come back as positive for Turner's Syndrome - a genetic disorder associated with short stature, a webbed neck and infertility. Eventually, after weeks of consulting foetal-medicine specialists, invasive diagnostic tests and countless sleepless nights contemplating a termination, they finally discovered that their child was fine - the NIPT had given them a 'false-positive' result, leaving a legacy of distress and health anxiety in its wake.

Like all parents, I wanted a healthy child but, perhaps uncharac-teristically for me, I decided to release control and allow nature to do its thing. The decision was ours as a couple, but it was one that could have been entirely different at another time, in a different pregnancy or with a more severe genetic disorder. Dads I've met who have been through a termination of pregnancy after genetic testing have had a variety of experiences. Many felt that, as a couple, they made absolutely the right choice given the information available and their personal circumstances. Others look back and reflect on whether they might have done things differently a second time around. Nobody ever said parenting was easy.

What Women Want

DO discuss what you would do if a screening test showed a high risk of an abnormality, including how you both feel morally about abortion, before undergoing the tests.

DON'T freak out completely if your partner's screening indicates that she's in a high-risk category. She'll need your support more than ever, with a cool head to help her make decisions.

7

Penis

How, where and when this guy fits in

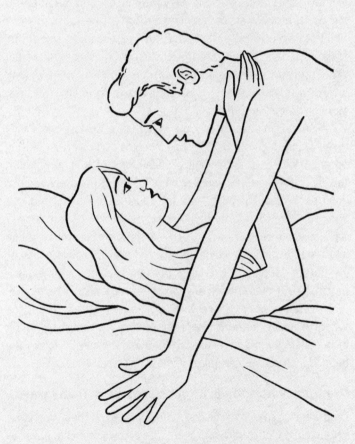

FROM THE DOCTOR

No matter how your partner became pregnant, this journey started with sex, and you've probably been wondering what the sexual forecast is going to look like while your partner is pregnant and, perhaps even more concerningly, after birth too. So, are there any rules and what is the temperature between the sheets going to look like over the trimesters? Before I'm accused of stereotyping men by having a whole chapter on sex in pregnancy, I should say that I regularly see women who sheepishly come to find out whether or not they can have sex during pregnancy. Man or woman, we all want to know, so let's get down and dirty with the questions that everyone wants the answers to, but many are too embarrassed to ask.

First, the brilliant news is that for most couples, sex during pregnancy is completely safe. If your partner is having an uncomplicated pregnancy, there's absolutely no reason why you shouldn't have sex as much as she – with enthusiasm from you – desires. More on that bit to come.

In some circumstances, your healthcare professionals may recommend that your partner has a period of 'pelvic rest' during pregnancy – this is really medical speak for no sex. It may be that this is just for a defined time period or for the entire pregnancy, so don't beat about the bush – ask the specifics of what is and isn't allowed. They won't be embarrassed to discuss it – they do it every day – so you shouldn't be afraid to ask. Reasons that you might be advised to avoid sex include a history of previous miscarriage or premature labour, a low-lying placenta (placenta praevia) – particularly if there's been any bleeding – or a history of cervical incompetence, where the cervix can open prematurely during the second trimester without other signs of labour, putting baby at risk of infection. So, if you're advised to abstain from sex, follow the medics' instructions carefully – if you aren't, then crack on.

Pregnancy hormones affect sex drive in many ways

Even when couples have no restrictions placed on their pregnancy lovemaking, it goes without saying that being allowed to have sex is very different from actually wanting it and this is where many people come unstuck. Let's start with your partner, because after all, if she doesn't want to have sex, then that's where the conversation starts, and, pretty swiftly, ends.

During the first trimester, some women find their sex drive soars. Pregnancy hormones can have an aphrodisiac-like effect and some women report a sex drive like they have never previously known. The increased blood supply to the pelvis, particularly the vagina and clitoris, can heighten sensation and arousal, so much so that some women report experiencing orgasm for the first time or significantly heightened sexual experiences compared to their non-pregnant sex. As with all sex, physical and psychological factors are as intricately entwined as the copulating couple. For those for whom the process of becoming pregnant has been challenging, with constant period-app checking and regular urinating onto ovulation sticks and a sex schedule that's more like a bus timetable than a spontaneous gesture of love and attraction, the sheer relief of having un-calculated sex can instantly restore the passion.

So that's one end of the spectrum and you might be thinking that this sounds ideal. But a soaring sex drive and new-found orgasms are not the norm for many pregnant women. These women report no interest in sex whatsoever, particularly during the first trimester. Add this to the other symptoms of early pregnancy – nausea, exhaustion and emotional turmoil – and you can quickly see how any sexual desire may vanish completely, no matter how much love and attraction your partner may feel towards you. The increased pelvic blood flow that improves sex for some can make other women feel uncomfortable down below during sex and further kill the sexual flame. Couples also often worry that sex during the early stages of pregnancy may increase the risk of miscarriage. There's no evidence that in uncomplicated pregnancies having sex will cause your partner to miscarry.

There's really no way of telling which way things are going to go and, like most of pregnancy, it's a rollercoaster that can change quickly with time. So, hold tight and communicate carefully. The good news is that for many, the arrival of the second trimester brings significant changes and sexual desires return once more.

Your own concerns

While your partner may or may not be wanting to have sex, there's a huge misconception that as men, we are always 'up for it'. It's very common for male partners of pregnant women to have concerns about sex during pregnancy. And no, this isn't normally related to your partner's ever-changing body shape. While any change can take some getting used to, many men find the physical changes of pregnancy highly attractive. In fact, it's often the woman herself who, despite heaps of reassurance, may be feeling insecure or lacking in confidence as a result of the changes her body is going through. For most men, reluctance arises from the psychological impact of having sex with a pregnant partner and, as we know all too well, anxiety does nothing for erections or libido.

Let's dispel some of the concerns that may be weighing rather too heavily on your mind. First up, if you've been given the green light for sex, or rather not been told to hold off, you're not going to cause any harm to your unborn child. Dads often ask about the potential for them to cause physical damage to the baby during sex. 'Will I be "hitting" my baby when I'm having sex', or, 'Am I damaging its head?'. Remember, your baby is safely contained within the tough membranes of the amniotic sac, which in turn is protected by the muscular wall of the uterus. Your penis will only ever remain within the vagina – no matter how big it may or may not be – and it cannot enter the uterus or damage baby in any way.

Many men report a strange feeling, or psychological concern, that having sex with somebody who is pregnant feels somehow different. It may be the thought of their offspring 'knowing' what's going on, or the thought that the baby might be in some way 'watching', that men find a turn-off. This is of course not the case. Your unborn child is blissfully unaware of what is going on as they reside snugly inside your partner's uterus. Be careful with anxieties such as this as pregnant women can mistake your reluctance for lack of interest due to her changing physical appearance. Careful reassurance and frank discussion about any concerns you may have about sex during pregnancy will help to break this potentially destructive cycle. If you are able to share all of your concerns as a couple in an open and fun way, you'll find the romance soon returns.

In the later stages of pregnancy, many dads worry that sex may bring on early labour. This myth isn't helped by the common advice given to couples as the due date approaches to have sex to help speed things along (more on that in Chapter 11). Semen contains the hormone prostaglandin, which, in very high doses – much greater than the small amount contained in semen – can be used by your healthcare team to bring on, or 'induce', labour. There's no evidence to suggest that sex will bring on labour before the body is naturally ready to start the process, so another unfounded worry dispelled. For uncomplicated pregnancies, sexy time won't bring on baby time – relax.

It's not just mums who feel the effects of hormones changing their sex drive during pregnancy. Doctors are beginning to understand more about the hormonal changes that take place in dads-to-be. The hormone prolactin has been found to increase as birth approaches and is thought to be associated with an increase in responsiveness to the cry and needs of your baby. Interestingly, levels of the male sex hormone testosterone fall around the time of birth, and with this, men may find their sex drive also decreases. It's thought that this may be a developmental response to encourage men to stay and nurture their family rather than to leave them in search of another mate. Whatever the truth, biology may well be involved with your changing sexual appetite too.

Talk and listen to each other

When you're both in the zone and have cast aside your pregnancy-related physical and psychological anxieties, what's the reality going to be? Pregnancy hormones may lead to an increase in vaginal secretions and depending on what you're up to you may notice a change in both their smell and taste. The increased lubrication may change the sensation both you and your partner experience during penetrative sex; some will love it, others may find it less stimulating than before. Sometimes hormonal changes mean there isn't enough lubrication, so if everything's a bit uncomfortable and dry it's perfectly safe to use a water-based lubricant to smooth things along.

Beware of the boobs. Forewarned is forearmed. Breast

tenderness, particularly in the first trimester, may well mean your partner doesn't want you going anywhere near them – for some that will be a huge disappointment as the ever-increasing size makes them increasingly tantalizing. Be guided by your partner and as pregnancy progresses, especially in the third trimester, don't be surprised if nipple stimulation during sex leads to a discharge of a small amount of early milk, called colostrum. An entertaining surprise and best to just laugh about together rather than focus on the bizarre reality that you may just have inadvertently breastfed from your partner.

As you reach the final weeks of pregnancy sex, it's worth considering some of the new symptoms that your partner may experience. Apart from the potential change in sensation, orgasm may be followed by some light, cramping, pelvic or abdominal pain. The increase in blood flow at orgasm can actually promote some very mild uterine contractions. These aren't dangerous and are completely normal, but can be uncomfortable, so a bit of post-coital lower back massage may come in handy here. However, if your partner experiences any bleeding after sex, or any cramping pains that don't settle on their own, she needs to contact her healthcare team. It may be nothing to worry about but shouldn't be ignored. The changing blood flow at the time of orgasm can also cause baby's movements to increase or decrease. Both are normal and as long as normal foetal movements return shortly afterwards, there's no need for alarm – and no, it's not your baby protesting about what mum and dad have just been up to.

Is there any infection risk?

It's clearly vital to avoid passing any infection to your baby as they're nestled in your partner's uterus. The baby is protected by the amniotic sac, uterus and a mucus plug that blocks the cervix, or neck of the uterus, so there's no risk from normal vaginal sex. If, however, you and your partner are having anal sex, be careful about following this with vaginal sex. Bacteria from faeces may enter the vaginal tract, which can put your baby at increased risk. If either you or your partner are having unprotected sex with other people around the time of pregnancy, there is a risk of passing on sexually transmitted infections. As with all sexual health advice, barrier contraceptive methods, such as condoms, should be used to prevent the spread of infection and any symptoms should be quickly investigated and treated by a healthcare professional.

If, as the birth approaches, your partner's waters break, your baby will no longer be protected by the amniotic sac that for 40 odd weeks has kept infection at bay. You'll be advised to abstain from sex, but from that moment forward, sex will probably be the last thing on either of your minds anyway. What is probably weighing heavily on your mind is whether you and your partner will ever want to return to sex again after the birth. Hold your horses, of course you will and we'll discuss exactly when and how once we've welcomed baby-you into the world.

FROM THE DAD

Getting a group of men talking, honestly, about their sexual experiences is normally a challenge. But the groups of new dads I've talked to have surprised me with their honest and open approach to the topic. The occasional beer may have played a part but, in reality, I think having a baby gives sex a different perspective. From the outset there's a change from the pleasure-seeking lovemaking to the evolutionarily purposeful baby-making. Once their partners became pregnant, most felt that the main change came from their partner's altered self-esteem. Changes in body size and shape made many women feel less sexually attractive even if the dads-to-be told them otherwise. During the first trimester, the nauseated hangover of morning sickness and my wife's utter exhaustion certainly dampened the flame in my relationship. But it didn't seem to matter; we both had a sense of purpose and maybe even sexual achievement that our bodies had 'completed' the act and conception had occurred.

As with many things, the second trimester brought with it happier times. I must confess though, long before the pregnancy bump was noticeable, I worried about the damage sex might cause. Despite having researched it extensively, and understanding the science, and knowing that it would do no harm, just the knowledge that my child was lurking within was always on my mind. Once the bump is visible, most dads said they worried about positions that might put pressure on their growing baby. However, they found innovative ways to avoid this. Upper arm and core strength were felt to be vital for dads-to-be, with 'the plank' providing enough of a gap in the earlier days, but with a more active press-up being required as the weeks passed and the bump continued to expand.

As the weeks progress, your partner may find lying on her back makes her feel lightheaded. The pressure of the baby on the major blood vessels in her abdomen reduces blood flow to the heart, giving it less blood to pump out with each beat. So, without providing you with a pregnancy-based *Kama Sutra*, I'll leave you and your partner to adapt your own individual style to suit her changing physical needs in private. I have no doubt your combined imaginations will be up to it. Leaking breastmilk came as a sexual shock to dads-to-be (and their partners). The overwhelming advice has to be not to focus too much on this. As with all sexual satisfaction, the psychology has such a great impact on the physical success and so most men decided to ignore the occasional nipple spurt in favour of keeping everyone's mind on the job.

Reassuring your partner about the love that you continue to have for her during pregnancy is so important. Most dads told me that, despite the fact that their affection towards their partners actually increased during pregnancy, their partners were convinced that they must be less physically attractive. Reassuringly, the dads felt that while obviously there were physical changes, they'd expected these and didn't find them the romantic turn-off that their partners seemed to be so preoccupied with. So, it seems that men may actually have been undeservedly stereotyped for generations.

What Women Want

DO make lots of time for intimacy and don't assume your partner doesn't want sex. Follow her lead.

DON'T be surprised if you find milk leaking from your partner's nipples and don't focus on it as you'll completely ruin the moment.

8

Genitals

Willy hunting and the 20-week scan

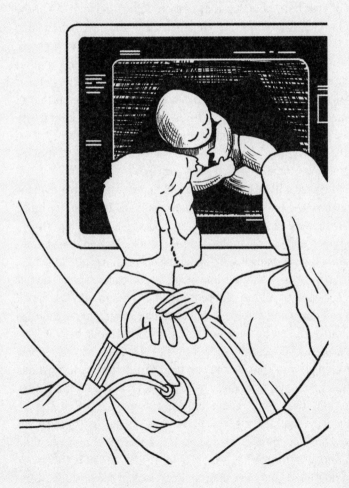

FROM THE DOCTOR

As you and your partner reach the middle of the pregnancy marathon, it's scan time again. Your partner will be offered a mid-pregnancy 'anomaly' scan between 18 and 21 weeks. This is a more detailed ultrasound examination of your ever-growing baby, and, if you haven't found out already through chromosomal testing, this is the first chance to find out the sex of your baby – if you want to, that is.

The main purpose of this scan is to take an in-depth look at all of your baby now that they're more fully developed. All of the major organs are now formed and in place and your baby's arms and legs are now more in proportion with the rest of the body. Even if you're not planning on finding out the sex, this is another pregnancy landmark visit that's worth taking time off work for, if at all possible. The scan can provoke anxiety for couples as there's always a risk of distressing news, so being available to attend with your partner is the perfect solution. All being well, it will just be a chance to have another peek at your baby, who'll be looking increasingly human as each week goes by.

The scan will take about 30 to 45 minutes to complete and is similar to the dating scan, but more detailed, as there's so much more to see. The sonographer will put some jelly on your partner's abdomen and use a handheld probe to look 'through' the abdominal wall to see baby inside; definitely no vaginal probe this time. Your partner's position is important so the sonographer can get a good look at all the different organs. The bed may be tipped up and down and she may have to roll into different positions to encourage baby to show and tell as required. Your baby will be measured again and the sonographer will look at the brain – now developing into specific regions for all of its different functions – heart, kidneys, abdomen, spinal cord, face and all the bones. Typically, they won't count the fingers and toes as it can be difficult to see them clearly at this stage. As well as checking out baby, the sonographer will measure the amount of amniotic fluid contained within the sac around baby, to ensure that it's not over- or underfilled, and have another good look at the position of the placenta to make sure it's not going to get in the way of baby's exit in a few months' time.

Normally the sonographer will be happy to talk you through what they're doing and show you the images as they go. Do ask questions by all means, but remember they're doing some pretty important checks, so try not to distract them too much from the examination; there will always be time at the end to talk through anything or show you any particularly good images for your ever-growing album of black-and-white ultrasound clippings. Most scans will be reassuringly normal, but if they do detect any abnormalities you'll be referred for further investigation.

To 'find out' or 'wait and see'?

Now when I said all organs are developing, that does indeed include the genitals. By now the vagina, uterus and fallopian tubes will be formed in a baby girl and the penis and testicles are present in a boy. But are you going to take the plunge and find out your baby's sex, or enjoy the guessing game for a little while longer? Although ultrasound scans are much better quality than they used to be, determining gender still isn't an exact science and occasion-ally mistakes are made. Whether you've decided you do or don't want to find out, let the sonographer know your decision at the start of the appointment. Occasionally couples spot something they wish they hadn't on the scan – in which case perhaps a career change to sonography is coming your way. Sometimes baby just doesn't want to play the genital-hunting game and is in a position that makes getting a good look between the legs very difficult. Some hospitals have a policy of not telling parents the sex of their baby and, if that's the case at yours, there are plenty of private clinics around offering gender scans for a small fee, if you really want to know.

Not finding out the sex of your baby has its advantages. Some people think it's cheating – like opening your birthday presents early. Probably the most compelling reason not to find out is to allow you to just enjoy the natural mystery of childbirth. Some women find not knowing the sex of their baby before birth a big motivator during the delivery. That excited announcement of 'it's a girl' or 'it's a boy' as your midwife passes the baby over can provide a final boost after hours of labour. The cherry on the cake if you like, and who doesn't want to feel a bit Hollywood now and again? Not knowing also keeps you away from gender stereotyping and filling your home with unnecessary amounts of pink or blue baby-related paraphernalia, and it prevents the 20 weeks of insensitive comments your partner might get if she does discover the gender: 'Oh well, next time you can try for a boy' or, 'I bet you were hoping for a girl'. People have an incredible habit of sticking their nose in where it's not wanted when someone is pregnant. Ignoring, smiling and moving on is always the best, and least upsetting, policy. And of course, not finding out removes that tiny, but still present chance of the sonographer getting the sex wrong and that awkward moment after delivery when you didn't receive quite what you and your partner were expecting.

On the other hand, now we have the ability to find out – pretty reliably – what sex your baby is, many people can't see why you wouldn't want to know as soon as possible. As a result, it's becoming increasingly popular to find out what sex your baby is at the anomaly scan. Knowing in advance helps with planning – and not just in choosing what colour to paint the nursery walls. Name selection suddenly becomes much more focused if you can ignore half of the baby name book and focus on just one gender. If either you or your partner has a strong desire to have either a boy or girl, you could argue that finding out well before the birth will give you time to adjust to what's been decided months ago by your genes anyway. In reality, once your baby is in your arms the stereotyped scenarios you may have been running through in your mind about playing football with your son or walking your daughter down the aisle will all pale into insignificance beside the utter joy of meeting the new arrival. Anyway, your daughter might be a top footballer and your son may want you to walk him down the aisle.

Whether you're in the 'find-out-now' or 'wait-and-see' camp, what's vital is that you're in it together. If there's a difference of opinion between you both as to whether or not to find out, this can make things tricky. Try to come to a unanimous decision. I've seen couples who've tried to make it work with one finding out and the other remaining in the dark. Inevitably, somebody lets something slip and it usually ends in tears, so I'd advise all in or all out. Your partner is carrying this baby, so ultimately best to go with her decision. If you've decided to find out, you can now set to work on the most creative way to let your friends and family know the news. From coloured helium balloons to personalized cards and reveal parties, the Internet is awash with creative, and sometimes frankly ridiculous, gender reveal ideas.

New symptoms for the second half of pregnancy

As your partner hits the 20-week mark, if it hasn't already, you'll most likely notice the pregnancy bump beginning to show. By this time, the top of the uterus will have reached the belly-button and the bump will grow by about a centimetre each week from now on. At some point between 18 and 20 weeks, your partner may start to feel the baby move for the first time; for some women it takes a little longer. Over time, they'll start to notice a pattern of movements throughout the day and it won't be long before you'll be able to feel them too. Inevitably the first few times you rush your excited hand to your partner's belly in an attempt to feel movement your child will get stage fright and stop completely. Keep at it and before you know it you'll be trying to decide whether you've just felt a right hook, a sharp elbow or the tiny foot of a future ballerina. Once your partner gets used to these routine foetal movements it's important to keep a careful eye on them each day. If she's worried baby hasn't moved for a while, things like an iced cold drink, moving around or the sound of music might stimulate things, but an absence of foetal movements or change in pattern might signal a problem with baby and should be discussed with your healthcare team straight away. There are loads of smartphone apps available to help you track foetal movements and build up a picture of the daily pattern.

The increasing bump size brings excitement, but also another collection of potentially unwanted symptoms. Back pain is common, as not only does the weight of the bump put strain on the back, but the hormone relaxin, which readies the body for childbirth, 'relaxes', or loosens, the muscles and the ligaments that hold joints together, increasing the risk of strains and sprains. Simple strategies can be really helpful. Sensible supportive shoes are a key first step; high heels should be avoided wherever possible. Sitting in chairs with good back support is important and using a small footstool to slightly raise the feet can be really helpful, particularly if at a desk for prolonged periods when working.

Relaxin has a similar effect on the ligaments that surround the uterus, particularly the round ligament, as well as those that support the bones that make up the pelvis. While this is a crucial part of preparing the birth canal to accommodate a baby passing through, it can bring with it the misery of pelvic-girdle pain. Gentle exercise and avoiding overexertion help, and a belly support can also provide welcome relief if symptoms are intolerable – but shouldn't be worn all day. These come in many different styles and designs – as part of clothes, belts or slings – and essentially support the belly, taking the weight off the aching joints. If simple measures aren't cutting it, check in with the healthcare team to see whether they can recommend further treatments such as physiotherapy.

Back pain, pelvic-girdle pain and a baby kicking away inside don't make for the best night's sleep for your partner. Combine that with her need for regular night-time trips to the bathroom, and you may find you're both getting in some sleep-deprivation training before baby has even arrived.

Recent studies have confirmed what we'd always suspected, that if your partner sleeps on her back during the later stages of pregnancy, this is associated with a small but significant increase in the chance of stillbirth. The weight of a baby-filled uterus pressing down on the major blood vessels that return blood to the heart through the abdomen has an impact on blood flow to the uterus, placenta and baby, so lying on the left side is the best position to sleep in. Of course, this is easier said than done. We typically move hundreds of times as we sleep, so don't panic if your partner wakes up on her back. Simply encourage her to roll over to go back to sleep. Using a pregnancy pillow – a bizarre, bendy, sausage-shaped pillow – can provide excellent pelvic, bump and back support as well as helping to keep your partner on her left-hand side. If you don't fancy shelling out for a new pillow, putting a regular pillow between the legs with another under the bump will do just as well.

More trips to the clinic

If your partner's pregnancy is progressing without complication and the scans have all been normal, the anomaly scan may well be the final sight you get of your baby before the big delivery day. Some clinics and hospitals do offer scans in the third trimester, and if any abnormalities have been highlighted, your healthcare team may offer further check-up scans as baby continues to grow. What's certain, though, is that your partner will start to have an increasing number of appointments with her healthcare team as the EDD approaches and it's important for you both to get a clear idea of the schedule in your minds.

So, what will these appointments involve? While they're an important opportunity for you or your partner to ask any questions about the pregnancy or birth as they arise, there are a few key tests that will routinely be performed so that the healthcare team can check in on both mum and baby's health as birth approaches. Your partner's blood pressure will be checked to ensure it's not higher than it should be and they'll also want to test a sample of her urine to make sure there's no sign of protein leaking out of the kidneys and into the urine itself. High blood pressure combined with protein in the urine may be a warning sign that your partner is developing a condition called pre-eclampsia. Symptoms like headache, visual disturbance and swelling of the feet, ankles, hands and face can also occur. The exact cause of this condition is still unclear, but if untreated it can progress to full 'eclampsia', which is potentially life-threatening, causing seizures in the mother and an associated risk of harm to the baby. Urine is also checked for glucose as sugar in the urine may be a sign that your partner is developing gestational diabetes.

The team will want to check that your partner is continuing to feel baby moving and will have a good feel of her tummy to check baby's position. As the weeks progress the midwife will take an increasing interest in this position. Ideally for a vaginal birth, by 36 weeks, the baby will be lying with their head downwards and facing your partner's back – but more on this in Chapter 10. Next, it's out with the measuring tape, to measure the distance between the top of the uterus (by now somewhere above the belly-button) and the pubic bone – the bone just above the vagina. Measuring this distance enables them to work out whether baby is growing appropriately and ensures that there's the correct amount of amniotic fluid in the sac surrounding baby. Finally, they may use a Doppler probe – a handheld ultrasound without a screen – to listen in to baby's heart. Normally you'll be able to hear this too, but don't panic if it takes a while for them to track down the heartbeat – depending on baby's position it can be a challenge to get the probe in exactly the right spot to pick up the sound. All the findings will be recorded in your partner's maternity record book.

Before you leave, your team should provide your partner with details of what to do if she experiences any complications or unusual symptoms as pregnancy progresses – there will be a list of numbers to call in her record book. Make sure you know where to find them as you never know when they might come in useful. If either of you are unclear about the backup and support available, be sure to ask.

FROM THE DAD

My wife says she always knew we'd have a daughter. I wasn't so sure but kept running through in my mind whether I'd be a better dad to a girl or a boy. I never came to any decision, but thinking about it really focused my mind on the prospect of becoming a father and what that really meant. I started to contemplate what was good about my own upbringing, what I'd want from my parents nowadays if I was a child as well as the different skills that we could both bring to the parenting team. One thing was for certain: we were both far too impatient to wait another four months to find out the sex of our child; if it was possible, we were going to find out at the 20-week scan.

After what seemed like an eternity of carefully scanned brain, bones, bowels and every other vital organ, the sonographer turned to us and asked if we wanted to know the sex. I think she had already seen everything she needed to give us this hallowed answer, but dutifully scanned around to show us the all-important 'between legs' view. When she uttered the words 'she's a girl', my wife simply said, 'I've always known she was' and I, rather less prophetically, asked whether she was sure there wasn't just a very small willy hidden away somewhere? I immediately regretted the question, realizing that I looked like a desperate modern-day Henry VIII, unnecessarily fixated on having a son and heir. This wasn't actually what I meant - though my mind had immediately flashed to the hours of my life I could soon be spending sitting on the 'dad chair' outside clothes-shop fitting rooms while my girl squad cat-walked their potential purchases. The sonographer gave me a disapproving look. I wasn't the chauvinistic testosterone-fuelled geezer my question had implied, I was just a doubting doctor wanting to be certain she hadn't made a mistake. I also thought that the discovery would unleash a world of girl-related product purchasing and that a wrong gender diagnosis could have been fatal - for the bank balance if nothing else. She looked me straight in the eye and vowed, 'I've never been wrong so far'. That was good enough for me.

As the bump started to become evident, I couldn't wait to feel the first kicks from our daughter growing within. For a week or two my wife thought she could feel some movements but laying a hand on her belly at the right time was tricky and whenever I did feel something, I couldn't be sure whether it was baby or bowel gently moving under my fingers - not quite the high-five I'd envisaged giving my daughter through the wall of her uterine cell. Soon enough, the fluttering became kicks and punches, though working out whether it was an arm or leg was almost impossible. Talking to the bump seemed a bit mad at first but combining the odd chat with a gentle massage and even the occasional song really helped us to bond from our two shores of the amniotic-fluid-filled ocean. There is scientific evidence that dads who talk to their baby and massage the baby bump find it easier to bond with their baby after the birth and they're also less likely to suffer with post-natal depression. The physical connection with your partner and the affectionate reminder that you too care for the ever-stretching abdominal wall and all that it's going to bring makes carving out some time in your busy life to focus on the bump together fully worthwhile.

It's a weird feeling knowing that one of your most incredible achievements is growing inside somebody else. Also, if you see that person every day, the changes are so subtle that they creep up on you almost without you realizing. It's only when you see a pregnant woman you haven't set eyes on for a few months that you fully appreciate the massive change her body is going through. There's always that, hopefully, internalized thought of, 'Wow, you're massive', before you proclaim, 'You look amazing'. I can honestly say there was never a moment in our pregnancy where I did anything other than marvel at the incredible physical changes Mother Nature had enabled my wife to go through for the sake of the continuation of our species.

It's easy to become paranoid that things are going wrong though. I'd often come home from work and gently enquire whether the baby had been moving lots today. My wife, being busy and fairly relaxed about the whole process, would sometimes say she didn't think she'd felt any movement for several hours, which sent me into a spin of anxiety and worry. Luckily, with a bit of concentration, the foetal footballing or ballet-dancing prodigy inevitably restarted her moves. One evening, I borrowed an ultrasound Doppler from work and, much like at midwife appointments, set about trying to find the sound of our baby's beating heart. Also, much like midwife appointments, there was a very nerve-wracking minute or two during which I gently readjusted the probe's position, with an ever-increasing sense of panic that the lack of audible heartbeat was not due to my poor skill, but because of a serious underlying problem. Whether you've bought your own Doppler to play with at home or are nervously waiting for the healthcare professional to find the heartbeat at one of your partner's many check-ups, remember that the probe has to be pointing in exactly the direction of the heart before you'll hear anything. If you can't hear a tiny heartbeat straight away resist all temptation to panic; the stressed look on your face certainly won't help the midwife find it any faster. Lovely as it is to have some earthly contact with your growing offspring, if anxiety is even vaguely running high, I'd put DIY Dopplers into the don't-try-this-at-home category and leave it to the pros.

What Women Want

DO discuss and come to an agreement about whether or not you'll find out the sex of your baby before you go for the anomaly scan.

DON'T ask friends and family opinions on potential names; make the decision as a couple.

9

Hands

Prepping for the big arrival

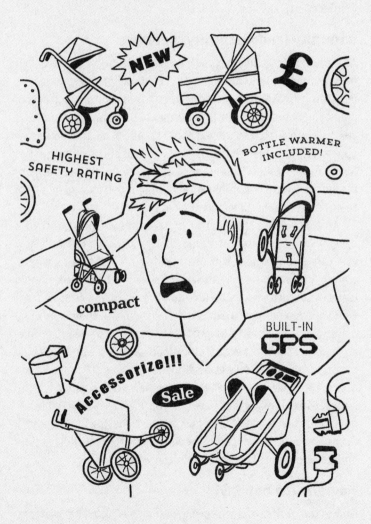

FROM THE DOCTOR

When it comes to baby-making, let's face it, your partner has really been doing most of the serious work, housing, nurturing, feeding and carrying the bundle of joy that's getting steadily closer to arriving. But while she's focusing on the biology, there's a whole host of life admin that you can get to work on – with input from your partner – to make sure that everything is in place for the imminent arrival.

Paternity (and maternity) benefits

As the bump's starting to show it's probably time for you and your partner to get all the arrangements confirmed for any maternity or paternity leave that you are entitled to. Check your contracts of employment for maternity or paternity benefits and find out what your statutory rights are; be sure to fill in all the necessary paperwork on time so that neither of you miss out on opportunities for financial support. Many employment contracts require your partner to inform her employer about the pregnancy no less than 15 weeks before the expected week of delivery.

As a new dad it's wonderful to have time to spend with your new family immediately after the birth, so consider carefully how you can arrange this. You are entitled to one to two weeks' statutory leave, but it may also be possible to add on some annual leave. Your partner may be able to have up to a year away from work, but don't forget to explore the possibility of shared parental leave, which has been a huge hit with dads who've successfully arranged it. The prospect of fatherhood can bring with it financial concerns, so now's the perfect time to get your affairs in order, taking specialist advice where necessary. Your partner will be awarded some maternity pay, but you may also be eligible for government child benefits or tax credits, so having the necessary forms and applications ready for when baby is born will save time and stress once life becomes a little more hectic.

How about a holiday?

Now is the perfect chance to think about taking a final relaxing, romantic child-free break away with your partner before baby arrives – a babymoon. It doesn't have to be the world's most expensive holiday, but time together away from your everyday world of home and work can help you to prepare for the big life change ahead without the distractions of your normal routine. It may be the last chance you have to go on a hassle-free break for some time.

If you're planning to go abroad, spend some time checking the travel regulations before you book. Flying in the early stages of pregnancy is usually safe, but check with your partner's healthcare team that they're happy for her to do so. From 28 weeks, most airlines need a letter from your healthcare team confirming that your partner is fit to fly. She won't be allowed to fly after week 36 if she's carrying one baby, or week 32 if she's carrying twins. If you are flying, remember there is an increased risk of blood clots forming in the legs when pregnant, so keep your partner well hydrated and moving as much as possible to reduce the risk. If you're thinking of sailing away on a cruise, do this early on as most cruise companies won't allow pregnant women on board after 24 weeks – no ship's doctor wants to be delivering a baby mid-voyage.

Bear in mind, too, that the risk of infection is higher in some countries. Malaria from mosquito bites can be a very serious illness for a pregnant woman and malaria zones shouldn't be top of your babymoon destination list. If it's unavoidable, your partner should contact her doctor to discuss which anti-malarial medications she can take to reduce the risk of infection. While we're worrying about mosquitos, Zika virus is another disease they can spread and this can cause birth defects, such as a small head and abnormal brain development (microcephaly) in a growing foetus. So, stay away from any moderate- or high-risk Zika areas.

Wherever you go, make sure you have adequate insurance in place before setting off. Healthcare away from home, particularly for a pregnant woman, can quickly become very expensive. Most standard insurance policies don't cover pregnancy and maternity-related issues if your partner wasn't pregnant when you took it out. Contact your policy provider well in advance to ensure that you have cover for anything unexpected that might happen.

Back at home

There'll be plenty of preparation to do here too. Planning where baby is going to sleep, preparing a nursery and building all the furniture that will be required is a perfect activity for a dad-to-be. No matter how good your partner's DIY skills are, all heavy lifting will be down to you. It's recommended that your baby sleeps in the same room as you or your partner for the first 6 months – day and night. There are loads of options from Moses baskets, cribs and cots to co-sleeping cribs that attach to the side of your bed, keeping baby within easy reach for those middle-of-the-night feeds.

Other gear that might come in handy includes a bouncer chair for baby to sit in during the day when they're awake so you or your partner can get on with vital life tasks. Carrying a baby in a sling, or what's now known as 'baby-wearing', can be a great way to transport the new arrival. Many dads find this a brilliant opportunity to bond with their new baby and enjoy being able to carry them hands-free. Slings and baby carriers come in all different sizes and specifications, so try to find one that works for both you and your partner and is designed for newborns and beyond. An organization called Babywearing.org arranges events at libraries and cafés that give you the chance to try before you buy – it's worth having a look online.

If you thought buying a car was a challenge, then welcome to the world of buggies. They're available in hundreds of different designs, with some useful and some completely unnecessary features, and price tags to make your eyes water. Choose a model that will fit with your lifestyle and think carefully about whether you want a light-weight, slimline, city run-around or a 4×4 country off-roader before committing to a purchase. Consider, too, where you'll store it, how heavy it is, whether it fits into the back of your car and how long it will last your growing child before you have to shell out for another one.

While you're checking out the car, getting a car seat is going to be essential if you're planning to drive anywhere with your new baby – even to take them home from the hospital. According to UK law, any child under the age of 12 years must travel in a car seat, and for the first year or so seats should be rear-facing. Here again, your local and online retailers will have a large range of options.

Some models have to be strapped in to the car each time with a seatbelt, which can be a bit tricky when you're carrying all the other baby-related accessories. Others clip directly into a base attached to fixation points in your car – worth considering for both safety and convenience, though check compatibility with your car first. Some can be clipped into a buggy frame, too.

A young baby needs to travel in a rear-facing seat, ideally in the back of the car. If you strap it into the front passenger seat, it's vital that the airbag has been disabled first. If you can't work out how to do this, and a garage can't help you, do not put your baby in the front seat; in a crash, airbags expand with enough force to kill a baby, so don't take any chances.

The all-important hospital bag

Your partner may well be starting to gather together the things she needs for her hospital bag, which will contain everything from labour comforts, clothes, cosmetics and nipple pads for her, to sleepsuits, nappies and wet-wipes for the new family member. It's best to have one packed and ready by 36 weeks at the latest. You should have one ready even if you're planning a home birth just in case your partner needs to be transferred to hospital in an emergency.

While you may be thinking that any involvement in the famous bag is well beyond your responsibilities or capabilities, I'm afraid you are very wrong. Of course, your partner is going to be making the contents decisions, but a top tip is to pack the bag together. On the big day itself, while your partner's in the throes of labour, knowing where to find the essentials is going to be fully down to you, so best to be involved from the outset. You'll also need to think about an overnight bag for yourself. As well as a change of clothes and a toothbrush, yours could include other items to make the stay more comfortable. Post-natal wards are kept at tropical temperatures for tiny humans so some shorts and a t-shirt can help keep your cool dad persona intact. A portable speaker for music and a well-selected birthing playlist can be invaluable for the hours of waiting that might ensue. Take along a selection of favourite snacks for both you and your partner – labour can be a hungry business. Throwing in a couple of extra pillows can also make the hospital stay much more comfortable. If you haven't slept a night on a hospital pillow, you may think this is unnecessary, but the familiarity and comfort of even a basic home pillow is fantastic both during and after labour. Don't worry about being judged by the delivery team when you arrive – most people arriving on the labour wards look like they're moving in for a few weeks. Don't forget to take the car seat in either if you're planning on bringing baby home by car. Some items will need to go in at the last minute, so have a list ready of the essentials that you'll need to throw in as you rush out the door.

Prepping yourselves for the big day

It's not just your partner who'll benefit from being in good physical shape for labour, birth and the start of parenthood. Supporting your partner in labour can be physically and psychologically demanding. Once the baby is born you'll find yourself carrying them, complete with all their accessories. So, you too will benefit from some time spent getting physically fit in the run-up to delivery day. A baby-related sprain or strain will be less likely if your core is conditioned and your biceps buffed. If you've ever tried standing up from a sitting position without using your hands, while carrying a child, you'll realize that a bit of core strength goes a long way. If fitness isn't normally your thing, now's the perfect chance to get in shape before any hope of a gym schedule goes on a temporary hold.

A good understanding of labour and your birthing options will help both you and your partner to prepare a 'birth plan' – your bespoke list of wishes for the labour and birth of your child. Reading this book should give you much of the knowledge you'll need but booking onto a course of antenatal classes is a brilliant way to increase your knowledge, ask questions and meet others in the same boat. There will be classes available locally, either run by hospitals or clinics or by external organizations, and finding one that's near to where you live is advisable. Not only will it make getting there so much easier, but it will also give you the chance to meet other parents-to-be in your area. This is not only useful now, but it's invaluable when you all have babies of a similar age too. Classes can teach you useful practical techniques, such as massage, for supporting your partner in labour, and provide a useful opportunity to discuss your birth plan with an experienced midwife or birthing partner; people often pick up vital tips from other parents-to-be. It can also be reassuring to discover that you're not alone with any anxieties you might have about becoming parents. Being prepared for what lies ahead automatically removes so much of that fear of the unknown, so go on, become a pregnancy and birth guru and the ultimate birthing companion for your partner.

FROM THE DAD

After scrolling through YouTube videos showing exactly how certain buggies would fit into different cars, it became blatantly clear that while we might fit the buggy into the boot of our beloved Mini, we'd either need to accept that this would be the only item coming on any trips with us, or do the inevitable, and find a more family-friendly car. There's nothing quite like being forced to replace your car as the first reminder of the financial implications of starting a family. If you're reading this knowing that your treasured supercar barely accommodates an overnight bag, let this be a gentle warning that although babies themselves are very small, their necessities and accessories are most certainly not. Space may well have to take priority over style and if you're thinking of having more than one child, going big early on with cars may save you a load of cash in a few years' time. I'm no car expert, so I won't attempt to advise on ideal models, but prioritize boot space, car-seat fixation points and safety if you're contemplating a pre-arrival car switch.

Even if you successfully dodge the car-buying bullet, you'll no doubt still find yourself contemplating chassis, wheel hubs and body designs of a different sort as the search for the buggy commences. A visit to the local department store was not dissimilar to a trip to a car showroom, with delightful salespeople eager to flog the latest all-singing, all-dancing buggy with its uniquely patented folding mechanism and modular design at an astronomical price. Talk of improved 'baby safety' really hits you where it hurts, and if you're not careful you'll find you could nearly have bought a car for the price of some of the designer buggies available. We settled for a slimline city model, which was perfect for roaming the London streets. However, a few months later an attempt at what should have been a relaxing stroll along a beach in Cornwall turned into a sled-pushing workout providing adequate training for someone wishing to enter a strong-man competition; the buggy was going nowhere and nor were we. One size certainly doesn't fit all when it comes to these machines and investigating the second-hand market is definitely worthwhile as many online companies offer refurbished versions of high-end models at much-reduced prices.

After a happy weekend spent assembling flat-pack nursery furniture, I breathed a sigh of relief as I inserted the final screw from the bag of what seemed like the whole world's supply of DIY fixings that I'd opened earlier that morning. But the preparation weekend was far from over; I still had two hours of 'pregnancy-partner yoga' to endure that evening. Now, I think yoga is a wonderful discipline and along with Pilates (taught in the right way), both are fantastic exercise for pregnant women, strengthening the core and helping with relaxation, but as a man with hamstrings so tight he can barely touch his toes, the thought of attempting any form of animal-related pose in public - downward facing or otherwise - fills me with stomach-sinking dread. Poses aside, the class actually focused on some brilliant massage techniques for dads to use on their labouring partners. Obviously, I was repeatedly reminded by my wife - through gritted teeth over the spa music and tea-lights - that I wasn't nearly as good at that particular back rub as the instructor who'd just demonstrated it on her, but hey, I was trying.

Next up were the antenatal classes that I was dreading almost as much as the yoga, having heard rumours about hippy earth-mother birth teachers preaching about the evils of anything other than a completely natural birth. In reality, I had judged too soon. Our teacher was exceptionally well informed and had supported hundreds of women through pregnancy and birth over the years, so gave us a very balanced view of all of the birthing options, and welcomed the dads to the party too. We hadn't planned to seek out a whole gang of new friends at these classes - and had been pretty against the idea of befriending people just because we shared a single common experience of successfully baby-making within a month of each other – but once the babies had arrived, the support and camaraderie of people in very similar situations was invaluable. And so, friends they became. Not a replacement for old friends and family, of course, but an amazing group that we didn't fully appreciate the importance of until later.

What Women Want

DO help to organize the nursery and take the lead on logistics and administration while your partner's doing the growing.

DON'T feel you have to buy all your baby items brand new – it can get very expensive very quickly.

10

Vagina

Different ways to get a baby out

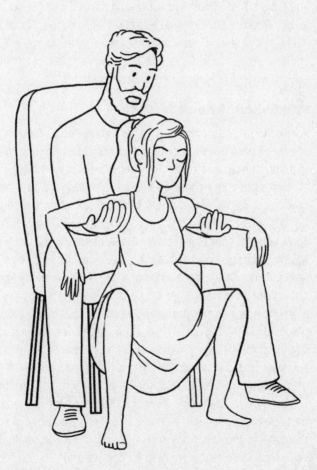

FROM THE DOCTOR

Now you're not only getting a daily view of your partner's growing bump, but can also feel your baby kicking away inside, attention has probably turned to not just where, but how baby is going to make its entrance into the world. Unless your partner unexpectedly gives birth in the supermarket or in the back of the car, you'll want to have a careful think about where the ideal place to welcome your new arrival might be. You can choose between having the baby at home, in a midwife-led unit or in a hospital maternity unit – if you have a high-risk pregnancy, your partner's care may need to be managed by an obstetric consultant and a hospital birth is more likely. You will also need to understand what all the pain-relief choices are and how they work. Knowing the options will help you both to write up a birth plan. So, what are they?

What about a home birth?

For uncomplicated, low-risk pregnancies, ask your healthcare team about the possibility of having a home birth. While this may sound like a terrifying experience that should be kept well away from the kitchen sink or the carpeted living-room floor, a home birth is a fantastic option for many couples, including first-time mums. You'll be fully supported by a team of community midwives who'll get to know you and your partner over the weeks leading up to birth and having the baby in the familiar home environment reduces stress levels. You can even hire a birthing pool to set up at home – the ideal opportunity for you to get hands-on, checking water pressures, electric pumps and ensuring you've got all the right tap fittings in place before the big day arrives. Home births are associated with a slightly higher rate of spontaneous (not induced) vaginal births and lower rates of medical intervention (for example with forceps or a Caesarean section) than the other options. Your partner can still have pain relief in the form of a TENS machine or gas and air – more on these later in the chapter – but she won't be able to have stronger pain medications or an epidural. Of course, you're further away from the hospital for help if a complication should occur, but remember that midwives will be there monitoring your partner and baby and would suggest a transfer to hospital if they had any concerns. They may even help you with tidying up afterwards and the benefits of not having to spend a night away from your own bed for both you and your partner are untold.

What's a midwife-led unit?

Also known as birthing centres or home-from-home units, there are two different varieties. Some units are 'freestanding' – not physically attached to a hospital – while others are set up alongside a hospital, but both are staffed only by midwives. They typically feel less medical than a hospital maternity unit; many have a spa-like layout and are equipped with comfortable chairs, bean bags and birthing pools. These units aim to move birth away from being a medicalized experience and remind couples of the natural process that birth truly is – so massage, aromatherapy, dim lighting and your music playlist will all be welcomed here. Pain-relief options include a TENS machine and gas and air, as well as use of a birthing pool. Again, your partner can't have an epidural here as they need to be set up by an anaesthetist (more later in the chapter). As with home births, midwife-led units have lower rates of women needing to have assisted or instrumental deliveries. If your partner is a first-time mum, doesn't want a hospital birth, but is uncomfortable about the thought of a home birth, this could be the option for you. As with a home birth, if the midwife-led unit is freestanding, there may be a delay in being transferred to hospital in the unlikely event of a complication, but when units are adjacent to an obstetric unit, a transfer can easily be arranged at short notice.

Hospital birth

The final option is the hospital obstetric unit – also known as a 'labour ward' or 'maternity unit'. All the bells and whistles are here with full-time midwives, obstetricians, anaesthetists and, if necessary, paediatricians on hand. Some women with low-risk pregnancies choose to give birth in a hospital as they take comfort in knowing that the full support of the medical team is available to them. For women with higher-risk pregnancies or where complications have occurred during the pregnancy or in previous pregnancies, giving birth in the obstetric unit may well be the safest option. Constant monitoring of baby is available, so any foetal distress during labour can be quickly identified and acted upon. All of the pain relief options – except possibly the birthing pool as some units don't have them – will be available to your partner, with anaesthetists on hand to insert epidurals, if required. Your stay will certainly feel more like a visit to a hospital ward and there's a higher likelihood of medical intervention during labour on these units – but often for good reason.

How do we choose?

This is not always easy. The best starting point is for you and your partner to ask your healthcare team what options are both safe and available locally for this particular pregnancy. Each pregnancy has an individual set of circumstances, so what worked magically for your cousin, colleague or next-door-neighbour's partner might not be what's best for yours. Anyone you ask advice from will offer their often biased or unfounded opinion, so try to keep the focus on what you and your partner feel is best, taking advice from the healthcare team into account. Many units offer tours for pregnant women and their partners, which give you the chance to see the facilities first-hand and meet the staff. Even if your partner has already set her sights on a particular place of birth, I still strongly advise both of you to visit before the big day itself. Familiarity with the surroundings, even just from a single visit, can be so reassuring when the time comes. Knowing how to get in, where to park, where the reception desk is and what facilities are available makes life so much easier when you arrive with a labouring partner. Far better to do battle with the car park, entry phone or poor signposting on a calm weekend in late pregnancy than when contractions are hitting hard and fast.

About the pain relief

You don't have to be a genius to realize that labour contractions and passing a baby through the birth canal and out of the vagina is a painful process. But it doesn't have to be. Thanks to modern medicine, there are loads of pain-relief options available to your partner. While few women would describe giving birth as comfortable, pain can nearly always be managed to a level that's acceptable. As a birth partner, knowing what's available, when and in what circumstances they may not be appropriate, will help you support your partner's choices and be her advocate during labour.

Let's start with the options that don't require drugs or medications; the first is one in fact, you! Encouragement, emotional support and reassurance from a calm and well-informed birth partner has a huge impact on a woman's ability to withstand pain and remain motivated throughout labour. A woman giving birth lying flat on her back, as so often seen on TV and in films, is rarely the most efficient or pain-relieving position to be in. Encourage your partner to try different positions that help to open the birth canal, like leaning forward, rocking gently or a supported squat holding onto your forearms. Learn a few massage techniques and you can provide relief for lower back and pelvic pain. These methods can be used wherever your partner chooses to have your baby. They are what you make them. My recommended gym workout wasn't just aimed at holding baby in the weeks to come; labour can mean hard physical work for the birth partner too if you're doing your job correctly. A warning note though: never complain that you're getting tired or can't carry on.

Whether in your recently filled birthing pool at home or the permanent high-spec model in a midwife-led unit, many women report huge benefit and pain relief from labouring – and giving birth – in warm water. Just because your partner decides she wants to use water for pain relief, doesn't mean that she has to remain confined to the pool forever more. She may find a warm bath at home during early labour helps with the contractions. Running a hot shower over her lower back or abdomen may also be really helpful. Being in a birthing pool not only eases the discomfort, but it also enables your partner to get into natural positions for giving birth, such as squatting.

Not all women who use a birthing pool for labour give birth in the water, so if your partner wants to get out before baby is delivered that's no problem. Equally, as your baby will still be receiving oxygen and nutrients from the placenta and umbilical cord at the time of birth, they can happily be born underwater without any issue. Warm water around the vaginal entrance and perineum (area between vagina and anus) also helps to soften and relax the skin, allowing an increased stretch as baby's head comes through. A water birth is for low-risk and uncomplicated pregnancies. The midwife will want to check baby's heartbeat regularly using a hand-held Doppler, much like they did at the antenatal check-ups. Any changes in heart rate might signal foetal distress and if the midwife is concerned about the baby, they'll encourage your partner back on to dry land pretty quickly. Labouring in a birthing pool reduces the chances of needing other pain-controlling drugs, but getting in too early can slow down labour, so most units wouldn't advise your partner to use the pool until it's well advanced and she's at least 5 centimetres dilated (about halfway there). There's more on this to come in the next chapter.

Technology is now very much on our side, so why not embrace that too? May I introduce the TENS (transcutaneous electrical nerve stimulation) machine. TENS machines, which can be bought or hired, have three or four adhesive pads that are placed on the lower back and connected by wires to a small handheld device that produces electrical impulses, the strength of which can be controlled by the person using it. The theory is that these impulses stimulate the body's natural pain-relieving hormones, endorphins, and at the same time partially block the nerves carrying pain sensation up the spinal cord to the brain. Some women find TENS very helpful in the early stages of labour, but there's limited clinical evidence to support its use once active labour has set in. TENS machines are easy to use, but I'd recommend having a go yourself at home before the big day – buy a few sets of pads to practice with. Starting early in labour seems to be the key to getting maximum benefit, and your partner can increase the intensity as required. The pads can get in the way of back massage and of course, don't take the TENS machine anywhere near water (baths, showers or birthing pools) – electrical impulses and water don't mix safely. Used correctly, a TENS machine causes no harm whatsoever to mother or baby.

If you've ever watched a film scene of somebody giving birth in hospital, chances are they were sucking on a mouthpiece as contractions struck. This device provides 'gas and air', or Entonox, a combination of nitrous oxide (AKA laughing gas) and oxygen that can be breathed in through a mask or mouthpiece. It takes about 20 seconds to have an effect, so your partner should start breathing it in just as a contraction begins – long, deep breaths work best. The sensation is different for everyone but it's similar to having a couple of beers back to back; it doesn't remove the pain but does make it feel much more manageable. Some women find it makes them want to vomit or feel too light headed, but as soon as they stop inhaling the side effects wear off almost as quickly as they came. Gas and air can be used as pain relief anywhere. The midwife will bring a canister to you if you're having a home birth. In hospitals and midwife units it will quite literally be available 'on tap' through supply ports in the wall.

If natural pain-relief methods and/or gas and air are not enough, the next step up to consider would be an injection of an opioid-type drug, such as pethidine or diamorphine. These strong painkillers can be injected into an arm or leg. They normally take about 20 minutes to work and the effects last anything between two and four hours depending on how much is given. Many women report significant nausea as a side effect, so the midwife or doctor may recommend taking an anti-sickness medication at the same time. As the drug travels in the mum's blood supply, it can affect the baby's breathing after birth if given too close to the time of delivery. It may also make the baby drowsy, which can make establishing breastfeeding more difficult in the hours after birth.

At the pinnacle of the pain-relief ladder lies the epidural. This is a specialist local anaesthetic that numbs the nerves that carry the sensation of pain from the birth canal to the brain, significantly reducing pain in most women. It doesn't cause the nausea or drowsiness that results from some of the stronger pain-killing medications. Being a specialist procedure, it can only be performed by an anaesthetist, so it's not an option at home or on a midwife-led unit. Anaesthetists are often very busy as they're required for many emergencies around the hospital including Caesarean sections, so letting your delivery team know early that your partner might want an epidural will help with planning and hopefully reduce delays. An epidural could be a good option for your partner if her labour is particularly long or painful, but they can also slow labour down. Midwives generally advise against having an epidural too early and may also suggest avoiding one in the later stages if your partner is ready to start pushing. If things are too numb during the pushing phase of labour, or second stage, it may be difficult for your partner to push baby out. There's a higher risk of assisted delivery in women who have epidurals, too.

Here's what the clever anaesthetists do to get the epidural in place. First, a thin plastic tube, or cannula, will be inserted using a needle into a vein in your partner's arm or hand. This 'drip' enables the medical team to give fluids into the vein. Epidurals can cause a drop in blood pressure, so having some extra fluid on board will help to counteract this. Your partner will then be asked to sit on the edge of the bed leaning forwards to 'round' her back and to stay as still as possible. You'll be key in helping here. If your partner's moving around too much, it could be too dangerous for the anaesthetist to insert a needle so close to the spine; luckily, most women are able to remain still for long enough to get the job done. The anaesthetist will clean your partner's back and numb the skin over the affected area in the lower back with a small injection of local anaesthetic. A needle is then passed between the vertebrae – not as gruesome as it sounds – into a space around the nerves of the spine. A thin plastic tube is then fed down the needle into this space and the needle is removed. Local anaesthetic, and sometimes pain-killing drugs like opioids, can then be injected down the tube to numb the nerves in the lower part of the spine. The tube is then connected to a pump containing the drugs, so the midwives or doctors can top up the pain relief when required. Your partner will start to feel numb from the waist downwards and her legs may become very heavy, making standing or walking difficult. This inability to move into different positions for labour is one reason that progress may slow once the epidural is in place. To try to combat this, some units offer lower-dose so-called 'mobile epidurals' that aim to keep pregnant women mobile during birth – an option definitely worth discussing with your midwife. Whichever kind of epidural your partner has, she and the baby will both require careful monitoring during labour to ensure there are no signs of distress. The monitoring of baby will be done using cardiotocography, or CTG. Two large belts are strapped around the bump with a disc attached to each: one measures the baby's heart rate, while the other monitors the contractions. Together the results can be interpreted by your healthcare team to determine how baby's coping as the labour progresses.

Many women won't be able to pee once the epidural is in place, so a small plastic tube (catheter) needs to be inserted through the urethra (the tiny tube urine comes out of) into the bladder to drain the urine into a bag. This may need to stay in place for up to 12 hours after the epidural is removed, until the bladder starts to work again.

After the epidural has been removed, your partner may notice some lower back discomfort that will normally settle after 24 hours. Around one in 100 women will have a headache afterwards, as fluid that surrounds the spine and brain may leak out from where the needle is inserted. These headaches normally settle, but if they don't a procedure can be performed to patch over the leak with a few drops of your partner's own blood.

So, while an epidural may sound appealing in terms of the pain relief it provides, it's not without its medical accessories and side effects, and all the tubes and cables can make your partner feel far more restricted during labour. As with all pregnancy-related decisions, the balance of risks and benefits has to be weighed up carefully, prioritizing a happy and healthy experience for both mum and baby.

The right way down

In the last weeks of pregnancy, the healthcare team will be taking an increasing interest in the baby's position in the uterus. Ideally, for vaginal birth, your baby will be in a head-down position, looking towards your partner's back with the back of their head (occiput) pointing towards your partner's tummy.

But just like big humans, the little ones don't always behave quite as they should. Some babies will be lying sideways (known as transverse) and some will be lying in a bum-down or feet-first position (known as breech). Most babies move into a head-down position before 36 weeks of pregnancy, but 3-4 per cent remain in a breech or transverse position. Delivering babies who aren't head-down is much more difficult and can put them at increased risk, so if the little shifter hasn't moved into the right position by 36 weeks, the healthcare team may offer a procedure called external cephalic version, or ECV, a process in which an obstetrician or midwife attempts to manipulate mum's abdomen to encourage the baby to move into the head-down position. It's always done in a hospital and it can be uncomfortable but it works in 50-70 per cent of cases. If successful, your partner will be able to have a safer vaginal birth. Some units will allow vaginal births of breech babies in certain circumstances, but be sure that the risks have been properly explained to you and your partner and that the doctors and midwives involved have experience in delivering breech babies vaginally. If ECV isn't successful and the baby remains in a breech or transverse position, your partner will be offered a planned Caesarean section.

FROM THE DAD

Being the scientist in our duo, I confess to being very sceptical when my wife said she'd like to try hypnobirthing to assist her with labour and birth. With visions of stage hypnosis shows and fully grown men dancing around like chickens, seemingly having lost control of their faculties, I couldn't imagine how this would fit in amidst a world of birthing pools, gas and air or even Caesarean sections. But I wasn't the one who'd soon be passing a baby out through my vagina, so I agreed to support her decision and was very pleasantly surprised. Hypnobirthing, for the uninitiated, is a change of mindset combined with meditation and deep-breathing exercises designed to help increase relaxation and reduce anxiety. Rest assured, there's no loss of consciousness or control or a sudden belief in your ability to fly - it's really a form of mindfulness for pregnancy. You and your partner can either learn the techniques on a course or by using online videos or audio tracks. Contractions are re-named 'surges' and the whole outlook on labour is moved away from a scary, painful process towards a highly productive and progressive experience that brings you ever closer to meeting your baby. Following the breathing regimes and listening to the soothing voice of the meditation track with its gentle sound of waves lapping on the shore isn't necessarily going to reduce the chances of complications during labour, but if it can help your partner to relax, reduce adrenaline and allow our birthing friend the hormone oxytocin to flow, I'd say it's worth a try. At worst, it's a good way to pass the many potentially infuriating hours of labour.

Now if bump massaging, leg rubbing and joining in on the hypnobirthing relaxation isn't enough activity for a dutiful dad-to-be to get involved with, and you really fancy getting your hands dirty, there's always perineal massage to consider. There's some research to suggest that massaging the perineum, the area between the bottom of the vaginal opening and the anus (back passage), from 34 weeks onwards, reduces the risk of tears or the need for episiotomy, and therefore pain, following vaginal delivery. Your partner can either do this herself, ideally daily or every other day, or, with her permission, you could learn yet another 'massage' skill. I will warn you upfront that this is not the most sexual of experiences, but it did feel like a truly practical 'workout' that I was able to help with that may reduce the risk of problems down the line. It basically involves a gentle stretching of the vagina and perineal skin. It's easiest with your partner lying comfortably on her back propped up with pillows, with knees slightly bent and out to the side. Using plenty of unscented natural oil, like olive, sunflower or grapeseed oil, gently insert one or two fingers 3-4cm into the vagina and apply gentle pressure down towards the anus while at the same time moving your fingers outwards towards her thighs. It's going to feel weird for both of you and may be uncomfortable for your partner at first. Our ritual, for want of a better word, was to combine the massage session with a hypnobirthing track, using the breathing and relaxation techniques to help with the discomfort - a very mild form of birthing practice. You too can now become a perineal personal trainer; what a highlight for the CV.

Writing our birth plan

Once we'd carefully considered all the options for labour and birth, we sat down together with a paper and pen to write a birth plan. It's recommended that your partner writes down her plans for the birth so that anyone involved in her care when the time comes can quickly grasp a good understanding of her wishes. Dads should very much be involved as you're likely to be your partner's main advocate during labour and birth, so knowing her preferences is important. There are two golden rules for birth plans. First, keep it simple. It should be a quick summary - two sides of A4 paper max - no-one has time to read a whole book of wishes, dreams and specifications of exactly which colour hat your baby should wear on entry into the world. Secondly, it's only a plan and all plans should be flexible, with both of you remaining open-minded about how things may need to change even at the last minute to adapt to circumstances outside of your control. Don't let your partner fixate on one path only, as inevitably things never go quite as planned. Flexibility and open-mindedness will reduce the risk of feelings of failure kicking in if the plan isn't quite executed with the military precision originally intended. Whatever happens, the priority in any birth should always be a healthy mum and a healthy baby.

There are loads of birth plan templates available online to guide you through the different choices, but here is a list of some of the things you can discuss and include to make life a bit easier. If anything doesn't make sense, the next chapter should help you make an informed decision about your options.

- Decide who your partner wants present at the birth (birth partner) and whether that will be different if she ends up needing an assisted birth (forceps or ventouse, or Caesarean section).

- Which pain-relief options she's open to, including the order in which she'd like to try them. Don't forget massage and hypno-birthing breathing.

- What position would your partner like to adopt for labour and birth? Would she like to use a birthing pool, birthing ball or a relaxed mat and bean-bag style setup?

- Do you want your baby monitored during labour and if so how? Options include handheld Dopplers or more careful monitoring with the CTG machine. Remember that some methods of pain relief and delivery require constant monitoring for safety reasons.

- Are you going to be the one cutting the cord or are you leaving that to the medical team? And do you want to delay cord clamping until it stops pulsating?

- Does your partner want an active or passive (natural) third stage of labour (delivery of the placenta)? Under what circumstances would she change her mind at the time?

- Who's going to have skin-to-skin following different delivery methods? Try to find some time for dad skin-to-skin too!

- How will your baby receive vitamin K after birth - by injection or oral drops?

- What will you do if either your partner or baby is unwell after birth? If your baby needs to be taken to the special care baby unit (SCBU) would you go with them, or remain with your partner? Who else could you call in if you needed further support?

Once you've got your succinct birth plan down, stick it in the front of your partner's maternity notes, so it's sure to make it to the hospital in the inevitable chaos of the labour dash.

What Women Want

DO understand all the options for the birth so you know what's available and can be an advocate for your partner's wishes during labour and the delivery.

DON'T be surprised when things don't quite go according to plan.

11

Cervix

The labour explained

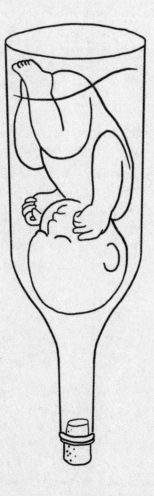

FROM THE DOCTOR

After around 40 weeks of waiting, the 'big day' is finally here. Nobody knows for sure what kick-starts labour, but understanding what to expect as things progress and what options are available is going to help ease the fear when the time comes. Remember though a 'term' baby is one that is born between 37 and 42 weeks of pregnancy; if your partner is showing any of the signs of labour described here before 37 weeks, you'll need to seek immediate medical attention.

Labour is divided into three distinct stages. In the first stage a woman's body prepares itself for pushing the baby through the vaginal canal during the second stage – birth. The third stage is when the placenta is delivered. All of this makes it sound straightforward, but like most things in life, it's not quite as simple as it sounds – ask any woman who's had a baby!

Here's an anatomy lesson

Inside the vagina lies the neck of the uterus, or cervix. Now imagine a bottle of wine hanging upside down. The wine-carrying part of the bottle is the uterus and the neck, the cervix. Obviously, it's all much softer and less alcoholic than a bottle of wine but stick with me. During labour, the cervix opens to allow baby to pass through. It does this in stages: first, the neck softens, then it shortens – imagine the neck of the wine bottle shrinking down – and finally it begins to open, or dilate, until it's 10cm across and the baby can be squeezed through. Compare this opening up to the neck of your wine bottle gradually widening to allow more and more wine to flow through. The midwife will measure how wide, or dilated, the neck of the cervix is using their fingers to see how far into the process your partner is.

The first stage of labour is divided into two parts: the latent phase and the active, or established, phase. The softening of the cervix begins in the latent phase. This can take hours, or even days, and may be accompanied by irregular contractions. The active phase is said to have started once the cervix is 4cm dilated. At this point, contractions become more regular and the cervix should steadily dilate until it reaches 10cm, at which point it's wide enough to get baby's head through and the pushing of the second stage of labour can begin.

How will you know that labour has started?

There are several clues that the first stage of labour has begun. Irregular contractions with cramping abdominal pain or lower back pain may signal things are beginning to kick off.

Some women have a snot-like mucus discharge known as a 'show' that may be slightly bloody. This is the mucus plug from the neck of the cervix – the cork of the wine bottle if you're still on that visual. Don't panic if your partner doesn't see this, many women don't.

Your partner's waters may break. The amniotic sac protecting baby contains a large amount of fluid. When the sac ruptures, the fluid will then leak out through the vagina. Normally, this is much less dramatic than in the movies, where they often depict a huge puddle of water flooding the floor beneath a woman's legs. Often your partner will notice a straw-coloured or light-pink trickle of fluid coming down her leg and wonder if she's peed herself. For many women, this happens in bed at night so encourage her to use a sanitary pad in her underwear as that will enable a midwife to get an idea of how much fluid has come out. If you're not sure whether the fluid's urine or not, a simple sniff of the sheet or pad will normally give you all the info you need – is it an ammonia urine smell or a yeasty amniotic fluid? Who said the partner couldn't get involved? Waters can break before contractions have started and the majority of women will then go into labour within 24 hours. Much like the show, don't panic if there's no sign of broken waters; some babies are even born wrapped within their unruptured amniotic sac. So, no sign of broken waters doesn't equal no labour. However, once the waters have broken the baby is no longer protected from infection so it's important to keep the vagina and birth canal clean. Nothing (other than examinations by the medical team) should be going inside now – no sex, no tampons, no nothing. If there are no signs of labour within 24 hours of waters breaking, your healthcare team may wish to consider inducing labour as there's an increased risk of infection after 48 hours.

When to call the midwife?

Most women can remain at home during the latent phase of labour – in fact you may be sent home if you attend the midwife unit or hospital too early on. This phase can take a long time and it's often quicker in the relaxed reassuring atmosphere of your own home.

There are a few occasions on which you should contact your healthcare team immediately and they will go through these with you as you prepare for birth. First, if the waters break be sure to let them know straight away. As there's an increased risk of infection as time passes, they'll want to keep an eye on things, to make sure that labour gets started and that your partner doesn't have any signs of infection, such as a fever. Likewise, if your partner was diagnosed as being group B haemolytic streptococcus (group B strep) positive during pregnancy – a commonly occurring bacteria that can live in the vaginal canal – the team may wish to admit her for intravenous antibiotics during labour to prevent infection.

Broken waters should be straw-coloured or slightly pink, but if they are dark, brown, green or smelly, tell your midwife as this may be a signal that baby has done their first poo – known as meconium – inside the uterus and this can be a sign of foetal distress. Likewise, a tiny amount of blood is normal with the 'show', but if there's heavier bleeding or continued blood loss, this could be a sign of a problem and your team also need to know. If baby is moving less than normal, or the moving pattern has changed, or you or your partner need any other support in the early stages of labour, call your healthcare team.

As a partner, being alone at home with somebody you love in labour can be an intimidating and scary experience. Remember that you're supporting your partner and that the medical team will value your importance in providing that role. In turn, they are there to support you, either in person or at the end of the phone. So, if you're worried, call them and let them reassure you or give you necessary advice. They'll have heard all the stupid questions before, so nothing you can ask will shock or surprise them – if it's on your mind, let it out.

How you can help your partner

Contractions are caused by the muscular wall of the uterus constricting and pushing baby further down into the pelvis and ultimately through the birth canal. Many women experience small 'practice' contractions, known as Braxton Hicks contractions, particularly in the final few months of preparing. These may feel slightly crampy but shouldn't be painful and are completely normal as her body warms up for birth. Imagining the sensation of labour is incredibly difficult, particularly if you've never experienced period pain and cramps, but if you take a look online you'll find videos showing men having the sensation simulated by electrodes stuck to their abdomens.

While you may not be able to imagine the sensation, that doesn't mean you can't help. Labour's latent phase lasts on average 6- 20 hours for a first-time mum – but can be longer (and is usually shorter for those who've done it before), so a whole heap of encouragement, reassurance and patience is going to be required. Many of nature's mammals head off alone to a dark, quiet place to give birth, and simulating this may be helpful for your partner, though she probably won't want to be alone. Creating a quiet, relaxing atmosphere is often the best way to get through. Birthing a baby requires a load of energy, so preparing a simple carbohydrate-rich meal for your partner of whatever she fancies will get the calories on board before the contractions ramp up and food is the last thing on anyone's mind. Be sure to keep yourself well fed too. Nobody needs dad fainting in the delivery room because he's not eaten for the last 12 hours.

If labour kicks in during the night, encourage your partner to try to rest where possible between the contractions; saving energy will pay off later. If things get started during the day then a gentle walk can help things along and is a good way to pass the time. Get your favourite box-set on, or watch some comedy – anything that keeps the mood relaxed and the mind distracted. If she starts to feel uncomfortable, now could be the time to try running a warm bath or sticking on the TENS machine pads. Remember the different positions that might be helpful in labour like squatting or kneeling or even sitting on a birthing ball. Start warming up your massage skills too, but don't peak too soon. Encourage your partner to take regular toilet breaks; emptying the bowel and bladder allows more room in the pelvis for baby to move down and having a pee is easily forgotten in the throes of labour. Before the contractions become too intense, make sure all the final bits are packed into the hospital bag and have a last run through the birth plan together so you're both clear on your partner's wishes.

As labour continues, the contractions will last for longer and occur more regularly and at a greater intensity. For some, the bath or a warm shower may provide relief, while others will want the cool breeze of an open window and ice-cold drinks. Having a bag of ice available for early labour is invaluable, whether to cool the water or to put on the wrists and the forehead as things hot up.

When labour steps up a gear

Being able to recognize when your partner is entering the active stage of labour is important, as it's at this point that you should contact your healthcare team, and/or get the car, taxi or friend ready for the journey to the midwife unit or hospital. Labour's active phase technically begins when the cervix is 4cm dilated, but nobody is suggesting you put your fingers in to try to work out how far gone your partner is. Counting and timing contractions is key and thankfully there are loads of free apps available to make life easier. Simply tap the app when a contraction starts, and again when it stops, and it will do the calculations for you – even providing some smart-looking graphs and tables to show the midwives or doctors if you so wish. Have a practice with your chosen app before the big day arrives to make sure you're down with the functionality. The active phase of the first stage is said to be established when contractions are lasting for more than 45 seconds and your partner's having three or more within a 10-minute period. Don't become a slave to the stopwatch though; stressing too much over the timings can ruin the mood and slow things down. If your partner feels things are progressing, be guided by her and talk to your healthcare team for advice.

Once active labour kicks in, the midwife may ask if they can do an internal examination to see how much your partner's cervix has dilated. Some women prefer not to have these examinations, but they can be a useful guide to progress. Discuss this and the timing of any examinations with your healthcare team. A contraction just after an internal examination may be slightly more painful so be prepared to support your partner through it. This active phase of labour typically lasts 6-12 hours for a first-time mum and your healthcare team will be keeping a careful eye on baby's heart rate throughout. As things intensify, support your partner to use the pain relief she'd previously settled on and make sure you're an advocate for her, communicating her wishes to the medical team when she's otherwise engaged. If there are changes from the plan to be made, you may be in the best position to discuss these with the team and ensure that your partner's wishes are preserved as much as is safely possible.

As the first stage of labour reaches its end and the second stage is about to begin, a rarely discussed phase called transition occurs. Every woman responds differently, but it's often the phase that is responsible for the hilarious post-birth stories or the craziest moments of labour. Transition normally happens between 8 and 10cm dilatation. Some women become extremely emotional or suddenly feel they cannot continue with the birth – I've even seen women demand to leave the hospital completely. Others will be entirely in the zone, often only able to make unusual noises or issue, sometimes seemingly irrational, commands. As a birth partner, this is probably the single most important time to remain calm, reassuring and supportive. Never try to make sense of the behaviour. Your partner will get through it, so just be strong for her and remind her of the amazing progress she's making and how close you are to meeting your new baby. And if you come through unscathed, quietly congratulate yourself.

The birth itself

After what may seem like an eternity, the cervix will reach the magic 10cm and become 'fully dilated'. Now the second stage, or the pushing phase, can begin. After months of waiting, your baby is about to make its way down the birth canal and into the world for the very first time. Encourage your partner to keep mobile as much as possible, though this might be more difficult if an epidural is making her legs very heavy. Many women describe this phase as like doing a gigantic poo. Imagine passing a bowling ball and you may be somewhere close. With each contraction the healthcare professionals will encourage your partner to push, with a break for a rest in between contractions. Your encouragement here is vital, reminding your partner that with every good push, baby is getting ever closer to the exit. This is the messy part of labour, so if you're scared of the sight of blood, maybe take a seat or keep your eyes away from the business end. If you're not, and your partner's happy for you to watch what's going on, get involved. You'll have a ring-side seat at one of life's great miracles – and when it's your child, the feeling is even more special. But, if blood doesn't put you off, be warned, there may well be poo involved too. It's normal for the 'pushing-like-you're-pooing' technique to empty everything, including the bowels, so if you're partner's using a birthing pool, be ready to sieve the floaters away. You're welcome!

Hopefully it won't be long before you can see the top of baby's head peeking out of the vaginal entrance. If your partner wants to she can reach down for a gentle feel – sometimes this provides much-needed encouragement. As the widest part of the head comes through the vagina – a process known as crowning – the birthing team will help to guide the head through slowly. They'll apply pressure to the perineum to reduce the chances of a tear as the vaginal entrance stretches to let the widest part of the baby through. Your partner's breathing here is important. The doctor or midwife will encourage your partner to pant or breathe gently, to stop her overstraining and forcing the head out too quickly. Imagine blowing out the candles on a cake six at a time, then taking a deep breath. That's what she's trying to achieve and doing it with her can really help.

The wait is over, and your beautiful, if rather slimy-looking, baby has finally arrived. Congratulations! Newborn babies can look a little blue when they first enter the world, and they don't always start to cry quite as quickly as in the movies. Don't panic if things take a little bit longer than you imagined; the medical team will be keeping a careful eye. Sometimes babies need a bit of a rub to stimulate them to breathe for the first time on their own, and they'll continue to get oxygen and nutrients from the placenta until the cord is cut. If baby is healthy, the midwife or doctor will place them on to your partner's abdomen or chest, depending on the length of the umbilical cord.

Skin-to-skin contact in that first hour of life is a great way to keep the baby warm and comforted as they can still hear the familiar sound of the heartbeat that's been their soundtrack for the last 40 or so weeks. As long as there are no medical concerns, the team shouldn't need to take baby away during the first hour – measurements and weighing can wait. This is an important and special time for you to begin to bond as a new family and will also be an opportunity for your partner to try breastfeeding, if she wishes. If your partner has had a Caesarean section, skin-to-skin with her is often still possible, but if it's not, you're the next best thing. Get that shirt off or pop baby under your hospital scrubs for your very first dad cuddle. Inhale deeply; newborn babies smell amazing!

There's more to come

The umbilical cord needs to be cut and finally the placenta needs to be delivered – the third stage of labour. Historically the cord was clamped and cut as soon as baby was born, but we now know that there are benefits to delaying this. For several minutes after birth, the cord will continue to pulsate, pumping blood and stem cells into your baby. It's now recommended, if possible, to delay cord clamping until the cord has stopped pulsating or to wait at least 1–5 minutes. The increased blood flow to baby will reduce the chance of anaemia and has also been shown to help both fine motor and social skills, particularly in boys. This isn't always possible though. If your partner is bleeding heavily or baby is unwell or distressed at delivery, it may be necessary to cut the cord more quickly to speed up emergency care for mum and/or baby.

Once the cord has been clamped, it's time for it to be cut. One of the team will happily do this, but they'll often ask the birth partner if they would like to do it instead. They'll give you some special scissors and show you exactly where to cut – between the two clamps. There are no nerves in the cord, so neither mum nor baby will feel a thing. The only 'nerves' involved at this stage may be yours. Be aware it's quite tough, like a gristly bit of steak, so it may take a few goes to cut through completely.

The last thing to make its way out is the placenta, and this can be done either 'physiologically' or 'actively'. The placenta is a large, bloody and slimy cake-like object with a similar consistency to liver. Although the contractions that expel it may be painful, it's so soft that when it passes through the birth canal it shouldn't cause any pain. Delivering the placenta 'physiologically' means doing so without medication and there may be a wait of up to an hour before it occurs; the midwife will apply gentle traction to the umbilical cord as the placenta comes through. The advantages of a physiological third stage is that it's drug-free, therefore avoiding common side effects of the medication.

If the labour has been more complicated, your partner's lost a lot of blood or the healthcare team have other concerns, they may suggest an 'active' third stage. If so, an injection of the hormone oxytocin (sometimes combined with ergometrine) will then be given into your partner's upper thigh as baby is born, or shortly afterwards. This speeds up the delivery of the placenta and reduces the risk of maternal bleeding after birth. However, the medication may make your partner feel nauseous for a short time and she may even vomit.

Once the placenta is out, the midwife will inspect it carefully to make sure it's all present and correct. Retained placental segments or pieces of amniotic sac can lead to infection or bleeding after delivery, so they'll want to know everything's successfully been delivered. If you want a look, now's your chance. If your partner wants to keep her placenta to encapsulate (the placenta is dried, ground and made into tablets), blitz into a smoothie, or bury in a special place, let the team know before it's disposed of. You'll want to make sure you've also packed a sealable bucket or box to put it in. There's an emerging market of novel ways of eating or drinking the placenta after birth (a practice called placentophagy), but there's currently no conclusive evidence that eating placenta, in whatever form, is of any clinical benefit to a new mum.

What happens if things don't go according to plan

The three stages of labour described so far have been uncompli-cated, but what, I hear you ask, happens if there are complications? We've all heard birth horror stories, but remember for some unknown reason, people are much keener to recount bad experiences than to talk about the many excellent birth stories that happen every day. Of course, things may not go exactly according to plan and fore-warned is forearmed.

Let's talk tears and episiotomies. Once you've stop wincing, we should face up to the fact that experiencing a tear during childbirth, particularly if this is your partner's first baby, is very common. As the muscles and skin of the vagina stretch to allow baby's head through, they're often unable to hold the strain, resulting in a tear, usually involving the perineum. Midwives are now trained to support the perineum during birth to further reduce this risk. Tears are graded on a scale from 1 to 4, with a grade 4 tear being the most severe. Grade 1 tears are only very minor skin tears and often heal on their own without stitches. Grade 2 tears are common and also involve the perineal muscles, so normally require stitching by a midwife or doctor shortly after birth. Grades 3 and 4 are larger tears, as they involve the anal sphincter (the muscular ring that controls bowel opening), with the most severe grade 4 tears extending all the way through to the rectum itself. These will need repair with careful stitching, normally in the operating theatre where lighting, position and pain relief can be carefully controlled, and may be very uncomfortable for some time after birth. Women with grade 3 or 4 tears may struggle with anal continence in the months following the birth, but specialist physiotherapy and care is available to help them return to normal function.

If a baby is unable to pass through the vaginal opening without assistance or they're becoming distressed, the midwife or doctor may suggest performing an episiotomy – a small cut in the perineum – to help get them out safely. The cut is usually made at an angle to the right side of the perineum, so that it avoids the anal sphincter and doesn't increase the risk of subsequent anal incontinence. A local anaesthetic will be injected into the skin before the cut is made, so the procedure shouldn't hurt for those without an epidural. As a birth partner, watching this can be distressing, so this may be one moment to avert the eyes, particularly if you're squeamish. Once baby is safely on dry land, the episiotomy wound will be stitched up, much like other perineal tears.

If an episiotomy alone doesn't allow baby to pass through the birth canal, or your baby is lying in an unusual position or showing signs of distress, it may be necessary for a doctor to perform an assisted, or instrumental, delivery using a ventouse or forceps. Normally, an episiotomy will also be required to help baby make a timely exit. It's worth remembering that these procedures won't be done without your partner's consent. If the medical team feel it's necessary, be sure you're both clear on the reasoning behind their suggestion. If your partner is reluctant to undergo this, make sure you ask about the potential risks of not following their advice before coming to a decision.

A ventouse device looks a bit like a sink plunger. A plastic or metal cap, attached to a suction device, is placed on to the baby's head, and the doctor will manoeuvre the baby as your partner has contractions. Babies who've been delivered via this method often have a boggy swelling on their scalp at the site of the suction cap. This will normally settle on its own within a few days, but it can take weeks or months to completely disappear.

Forceps look like large metal BBQ tongs and are used to grip either side of baby's head. Again, the doctor will use them to pull the baby through the birth canal during contractions. As with a ventouse birth, babies born with the assistance of forceps will often have some bruising to the head or face, but this will usually settle on its own over time.

Delivering a baby by either ventouse or forceps can be quite physical. The doctors and midwives will guide your partner through the process, but she will need to continue pushing with her contractions and the doctors will coordinate their pulls with these. Rest assured they will have successfully done this many times before.

When vaginal birth isn't possible, another route for delivery has to be found. An obstetrician will perform an operation to remove baby 'through the sunroof' as it were – a procedure known as a Caesarean section, or C-section. This may be described as elective, or planned, if it's your partner's choice because, for example, she has a fear or phobia of giving birth vaginally, or if there are medical reasons, such as complications in pregnancy or abnormal foetal or placental position. An emergency C-section may follow a difficult labour, an unsuccessful instrumental delivery or foetal distress. Whatever the reason, this can be a daunting prospect as for many women this will be the first major surgical procedure they will undergo. Knowing what to expect will help you to support her and prevent any nasty surprises along the way.

A C-section involves an incision of about 10–12cm across the lower part of the abdomen, just below the bikini line. The cut goes through the skin, fat and wall of the uterus, allowing access to the inside, from where baby can be delivered. It's considered major surgery, but it's a common procedure for obstetricians to perform and they become highly skilled at getting baby out very quickly when needed.

Obviously, nobody's going to take a scalpel to your partner's abdomen without anaesthetic to prevent pain. Most C-sections are done under what's called spinal anaesthesia. This is similar to an epidural, but here a one-off dose of anaesthetic is injected into the spine at the lower back. This numbs the nerves supplying the abdomen and pelvis, so your partner won't feel any pain during the operation and will be awake throughout. If she's already had an epidural, this can usually be 'topped up' to have the same anaesthetic effect. Women often describe a strange pushing and pulling sensation in the abdomen – like someone doing the washing-up inside you – as the operation gets underway, but an anaesthetist will be on hand throughout checking that she's comfortable. The good news is that you'll be allowed into the operating theatre to be present as your child is born.

In rare circumstances, either in a time-critical emergency, or if your partner is unable to have a spinal anaesthetic, it may be necessary to perform a C-section under general anaesthetic – so your partner would be asleep and unaware throughout. Usually in these circumstances it's necessary to get baby out very quickly and because of the emergency nature of the procedure, partners aren't allowed into the theatre. Should this happen, you'll be updated regularly and as soon as it's safe to do so, the midwife will bring your baby to you for that first skin-to-skin cuddle while your partner recovers from her surgery and comes round from the anaesthetic.

If you are heading into the operating theatre

The first thing you'll have to do is get changed into 'scrubs'. Before you start feeling like a star in your favourite TV series, be sure to tie the drawstring on the trousers tightly. Being left holding the baby is one thing, but if your trousers have fallen to the floor around your ankles the shine will really be taken off those first few minutes of fatherhood. Also, tight-fitting scrub tops may show off your guns, but they won't leave room for skin-to-skin with your new baby, so go for a slightly bigger size than fashion dictates. Your partner, meanwhile, will be wearing a hospital gown with an open back, to allow the spinal anaesthetic to be injected. As with an epidural, the anaesthetist will first numb the skin of the lower back with local anaesthetic, before then giving the spinal anaesthetic. Nobody wants to watch their abdomen being cut open when they're wide awake, so a screen will be set up close to your partner's head and you'll be invited to sit beside her, at the head end, along with the anaesthetist. As baby is delivered, the screen can be lowered so you can both watch the arrival into the world.

Prepare for the operating theatre to be a busy place, often with up to ten other people present, including the anaesthetist and their assistant, a couple of obstetricians, a couple of nurses, a midwife and a neonatologist or paediatrician. The procedure takes about 45 minutes from start to finish, but baby will usually be delivered within the first 5–10 minutes and this will be followed by the delivery of the placenta. Your baby can normally be passed straight to your partner, unless there are medical complications preventing this. Most of the time is actually spent stitching up the uterus and abdominal wall.

As there's been some pretty significant cutting and stitching going on in your partner's abdomen, recovery from a C-section will normally take longer than it would after a vaginal birth. The wound will need to be kept clean and dry and your partner may remain in hospital for a few days so that any pain can be carefully controlled. Your partner might need help to sit up or walk around during the first day or so, and will need lots of help with household tasks in the first week. Make sure she has plenty of pain relief on board and avoids constipation or straining. Lifting your new baby shouldn't be a problem, but nothing heavier should be attempted. It's also important to avoid strenuous activity (including sex) and driving until the scar is well healed and the pain has resolved – this may take 4–6 weeks.

Having a C-section doesn't mean that your partner can't have a vaginal birth during future pregnancies. There's a small increased risk of the scar rupturing during labour, so women having a vaginal birth after C-section (VBAC) are more carefully monitored, but if desired, a subsequent vaginal birth can normally be arranged – though it's recommended women wait a year after C-section before trying to become pregnant again.

You're ready, so where's this baby?

With all this new-found, labour-related knowledge, you'll find the excitement and trepidation around the arrival of your baby sharply increasing as the 40-week mark approaches. By now your partner will be feeling very heavy, sometimes uncomfortable and you'll both be desperate for baby to burst onto the scene and into your lives. Remember the key 'E' in the EDD ('estimated' delivery date) is just that. Only about 5 per cent of babies are born on the 'day' itself so don't fix your sights on it too strongly. If you went for a job interview and knew there was only a 5 per cent chance of getting it, you probably wouldn't have high hopes. The good news is that most babies are born within the week either side of their due date. If your particular bump decides to stay put beyond the 40-week mark, try to remain relaxed and reassure both yourself and your partner that whatever happens, within the next two weeks, you're going to meet your baby. In fact, thought of another way, this is potentially the last time you'll have as just a couple for many years to come, so try to enjoy it as much as possible. Being relaxed will help the process along anyway, so get the box-sets rolling, go out for a meal or do whatever makes you tick as a couple – as long as that's not an ultramarathon followed by a buffet of unpasteurized cheese.

If you've made the mistake of telling all your friends and family the EDD, you'll soon start to receive advice from anybody you speak to about the best ways to speed up baby's arrival. Some will come up with the strangest suggestions you've ever heard and others will simply give you a look, which is code for, 'You need to have more sex'. In reality, there's little evidence for any of the 'natural' methods of speeding up or inducing labour. After millennia of trying, if there was a guaranteed way to get things started, we'd all be doing it by now – but here are a few of the commonly suggested techniques.

SEX Enjoyable sex and orgasm may increase oxytocin levels, the hormone required to get labour going, but the increase will be minimal compared to the amount given to medically induce labour. Sperm also contains prostaglandin, which, at much higher doses than in an average sperm sample, helps to soften the cervix. Having good sex at this stage, with a large protruding bump and all the feelings associated with being heavily pregnant, may be a challenge. Spooning or doggy style are the best positions to try if your partner's keen, combined with plenty of nipple stimulation. There's no guarantee it's going to help, but at best it might be an enjoyable way to pass the time until labour kicks in.

CURRIES The theory is that spicy food stimulates the bowel and, in some way, may also kick-start contractions. This is folklore rather than evidence-based medicine and seems very likely to have been dreamed up by generations of couples looking for ways to keep themselves busy during the final few days of waiting. Behind the theory is the possibility that a relaxing evening out, without the stress of cooking and with some good one-on-one time as a couple, may stimulate our friend oxytocin again. Going mad on the spice may backfire though if your partner ends up with severe indigestion, already much more common in pregnancy, so if she's not used to spicy food, go easy and build up slowly.

PINEAPPLE Fresh pineapple contains the enzyme bromelain, a substance thought to help soften and ripen the cervix. However, a pineapple contains such a small amount of bromelain that your partner would probably have to eat 6–8 whole pineapples to get any benefit. That's more likely to give her diarrhoea and indigestion than to turbo charge the uterus.

DATES One study suggested that women who ate 6 dates daily in the 4 weeks leading up to their due date had fewer prolonged labours and were less likely to need to have labour induced medically. The study was only conducted on a small sample of women and a much larger group would be needed to confirm the findings. Unlikely to harm though, so maybe worth a try if your partner can stomach the sweetness.

CASTOR OIL Much like a hot curry, castor oil is thought to stimulate the bowel and simultaneously give the uterus a nudge to start off labour. In reality, it causes severe diarrhoea and, in some instances, vomiting. This is to be avoided as diarrhoea and vomiting can lead to dehydration – the last thing your partner needs as she approaches the labour marathon.

RASPBERRY LEAF Taken either as tea or in tablet form, raspberry leaf has been used by generations of women as it's believed to 'tone' the muscles of the uterus in preparation for labour. Some recommend having it from 32 weeks in gradually increasing doses, building up to 3 cups of the tea daily by 37 weeks. It shouldn't be started after the due date, as stronger contractions may cause foetal distress. Before your partner starts brewing up raspberry leaves by the gallon, she should check with your midwife or doctor as some women are advised to avoid it, especially if they are at risk of premature labour, due to have a planned C-section or are having a complicated pregnancy.

MASSAGE WITH ESSENTIAL OILS Many midwife-led units now offer aromatherapy to assist with relaxation and pain relief in early labour. The scent of essential oils, such as clary sage, is thought to stimulate oxytocin and assist with contractions. Therefore, it's advisable to avoid these oils at home before 37 weeks, or term, due to the risk of inducing premature labour.

COMPLEMENTARY THERAPIES Acupuncture, shiatsu and reflexology are all offered, at a price, as solutions to bringing on labour. Many women swear by their effectiveness, but as yet there's no research or evidence to support this. That said, if carried out safely by a registered practitioner, they may be a relaxing experience to take your partner's mind off the waiting game.

Why and when is labour induced?

As the EDD date comes and goes, it's not just your patience that's under strain. A pregnancy that lasts more than 42 weeks is known as a prolonged pregnancy and most units will be keen to help things along, or 'induce labour', before then. The concern is that, as time passes, the placenta becomes less effective and there is an increase in the risk of foetal distress or even stillbirth, with a sharp rise after 42 weeks for first-time mums. Rates for stillbirth are still fortunately very small, with less than 1 in 1,000 happening between 39 and 40 weeks, around 1 in 1,000 at 41 weeks, but increasing to 2 in 1,000 by 42 weeks.

It's still not entirely clear when exactly is the best time to induce mums who are overdue, but most units will offer induction 7–10 days after your baby's EDD – at around 41 weeks. Induction isn't just offered to mums who are overdue; it might also be offered when the waters have broken and labour hasn't started spontaneously or in a pregnancy complicated by a number of conditions such as diabetes, high blood pressure or concerns regarding baby's growth or movements.

While you're cooking up curries and trying to figure out the most comfortably accessible sex positions, your midwife may have another suggestion. For uncomplicated, low-risk pregnancies, a membrane or cervical sweep will be offered at the 40- or 41-week appointment. This is a vaginal examination, in which the midwife passes a finger into the cervix (back to the wine bottle neck) – if it's open enough to allow this – and pushes the membranes of the amniotic sac away from the wall of the uterus. This is thought to stimulate hormones, such as prostaglandins, and for some women will help encourage labour to begin. The procedure can be repeated after 48 hours if it is not successful first time; many first-time mums will need more than one attempt to get things going. The sensation can be quite uncomfortable, often described as a sharp cramping period-like pain, and it's sometimes followed by the waters breaking or a small amount of a bloody mucus plug, or show.

If a cervical sweep doesn't start labour, a medical induction will be recommended. Of course, it's your partner's right to refuse an induction, but before doing so consider the significant increase in complications, including stillbirth, that can occur after 42 weeks. If you have opted to hold off and let nature take its course, your healthcare team should offer careful monitoring with regular ultrasound scans to assess baby, the placenta and its blood supply, as well as the amount of amniotic fluid within the uterus.

What does medical induction involve, you ask?

This is best thought of as a step-ladder of approaches, moving up to the next rung on the ladder if the first one doesn't work. Induction will normally be carried out in a hospital maternity unit and starts with insertion of a vaginal tablet (pessary), or gel containing the hormone prostaglandin. Back to the wine bottle analogy. The cervix, or wine bottle neck, which needs to soften, widen and open, is stimulated by the high dose of prostaglandins. This is a super-strength chemical version of the mini-doses of prostaglandin you've been donating from your semen over the last few days. For some women, it may be possible to go home again after the pessary has been inserted, but the team will usually want to see your partner again if contractions begin, waters break or you have any concerns. If this isn't successful, the next rung will involve inserting another dose of prostaglandin gel or pessary into the vagina, to encourage that wine bottle neck to shorten and open even further. Before delivering each dose, a midwife will normally examine your partner to assess her cervix and see how soft, short or open the neck has become.

If prostaglandins aren't helping, the next step is a drip containing the hormone syntocinon, a synthetic form of oxytocin. A cannula will be inserted into a vein in the arm or hand and connected to the syntocinon drip. This would be done in a hospital maternity unit and your partner will need continuous electronic monitoring with cardiotocography (CTG) to measure the contractions and the baby's heart rate to ensure that the hormone is not causing foetal distress. Contractions resulting from a medically induced labour can be more painful than naturally occurring ones so many women choose to have pain relief, such as an epidural.

Sometimes, the team will suggest breaking the waters using a small probe inserted into the vagina. This is known as artificial rupture of membranes (ARM) and can help to speed things along, but is not conducted routinely.

Even with hormonal induction, labour can still take 24–48 hours to become established and occasionally women still don't go into labour, at which point an obstetrician will discuss the options for a further induction attempt or even a Caesarean section.

Your partner may feel very anxious about the thought of induction, but rest assured that as many as one in five pregnancies in the UK are medically induced. Mums-to-be should be central in the decision-making regarding the timing and circumstances of their induction and will still have a full range of supportive pain-relief strategies available to them. However, it won't usually be possible to get into a birthing pool during labour because of the closer monitoring required. There is a slightly increased risk of needing instrumental delivery following medical induction, but before long, your baby will be joining you and ensuring this happens as safely as possible needs to be the priority.

FROM THE DAD

After weeks of anticipation, our EDD finally arrived, along with not even the tiniest hint of a contraction. After months of waiting, even a single hour longer seemed too much to bear, but days went by and there was still no sign. The midwife visits filled some of the time, and on each occasion, they looked at me as if to say, 'You're probably not feeding her enough curry or having enough sex'. We tried every suggested labour-inducer, even though deep down I knew there was almost no scientific basis behind any of them – even just an outside chance of speeding things up seemed worth a try. Wedding videos and romantic films were watched in an attempt to get the oxytocin flowing through her veins and yes, we both had a lot of curry – though rather worryingly, the owner of our local Indian restaurant had never heard of the theory that curry sped up labour onset; he informed me that all of his children were at least two weeks overdue – perhaps his curries aren't hot enough. After a week of waiting, my wife tried reflexology, but still not a peep. Dates were beginning to be set for induction of labour and it felt as though she might just remain pregnant for ever more. Going in to work each day was painstakingly frustrating. I was on tenterhooks at all times waiting for that phone call summoning me to be by my labouring wife's side. My birthday came around and we decided to abandon all attempts at bringing on labour in favour of an evening of celebration – dinner, a few drinks and a birthday cake, with the tiny morale boost of realizing that at least my birthday would not be shared, and therefore overshadowed, forever more.

The next morning, I was awoken at 5am by my wife, who thought her waters were breaking. A quick dash to the bathroom and a small slightly pink puddle on the floor confirmed that things were, finally, underway. No contractions as yet, so after a couple of hours of pretending to sleep in bed and failing miserably, off we went for a walk. Waters were still leaking onto a carefully placed pad and after several more hours, the faintest sign of cramping labour pains began. Initially, they appeared to be so mild that we could continue our walk, but by the time we neared home we were stopping every 5 minutes or so for her to rest on me as her breath was taken away by the contractions. Now it was time to put what we'd learned at all those antenatal classes into practice, but which to try first; could I somehow use the birthing ball, warm bath and TENS machine all at once? No - calm down.

During the early part of labour at home, hypnobirthing worked brilliantly. My wife was calm and able to breathe through the contractions. Occasionally one would be so strong that she'd panic and lose concentration on her breathing, but a gentle reminder from me to keep focused and some help to count the breaths soon had her back on track. I remember my suggestion that we try the TENS machine was met with a snarl, but anything seemed worth a go and she actually found it very helpful, squeezing the boost button every time another contraction gripped. Meanwhile, I was massaging her lower back with one hand and dutifully logging the contractions on my frantically downloaded app, and of course I was in regular contact with the midwives to let them know things were cranking up. After months of planning a pool birth, a quick trial in a warm bath told me all I needed to know. It seemed to settle the pain for a few minutes, but soon she was feeling nauseous and too hot, so out of the bath she came. The windows were flung open and, despite my protests at leaving her labouring alone, I was dispatched to the shops to buy a bag of ice. It's unclear why I felt the need to tell the cashier that my wife was in labour, but I got a pretty disapproving, 'Why-the-hell-are-you-out-buying-party-ice-now-then-mate?' look as I tore out of the shop.

Having just the two of us at home meant that there were no distractions and we could keep the environment calm and zen, but the midwife's arrival was a welcome relief. I was doing my best to remain as relaxed as is possible when the prospect of delivering your own child seems to be looming ever closer, but having another non-labouring human present was as reassuring for me as it was for my wife. A quick internal examination revealed she'd soared past the magic 4cm and it was time to head into hospital. To avoid parking issues, my mum had kindly agreed to drop us off at the hospital. Many dads-to-be have told of frenzied self-driven journeys to hospital or negotiations with taxi drivers to ensure they're happy to transport a labouring woman. If waters haven't broken by the time you're heading in, a towel and a large bin bag could save you an awkward debate with a taxi driver about his damp car seat on arrival – don't forget the hospital bag, extra pillows, the maternity record book and, of course, the baby's car seat (if required).

Somewhere between the car and the hospital lift, the contractions had become too much for my wife and, having been against the idea of anything other than some gas and air, once in the delivery room she announced that she needed an epidural. As is often the case, the required anaesthetist was caught up in an emergency in theatre, so another painstaking wait. My wife was dragging heavily on the gas and air; the contractions were now back to back and seemed pretty relentless. It's hard to just sit by and watch as somebody you love and care about so much is in such pain and discomfort. Gentle massage, reassurance and a reminder about the impending joy of meeting the new arrival helped a little. I think the period of 'transition' coincided exactly with the epidural finally being inserted. Unlike many of the dads-to-be I've spoken to, I luckily avoided being bitten by my other half and by now she was too attached to monitors and drips to abandon all hope and make a bolt for freedom out of the labour ward doors. The anaesthetist took the brunt of the abuse, but once the epidural had kicked in she received a huge hug and some Entonox-inspired words of thanks and adoration from my labouring wife.

After about 14 hours of increasingly intense labour, another examination revealed my wife was 10cm dilated and after a brief wait, it was time to start pushing. I fumbled around inside the hospital bag – yes, we'd packed it together, but finding the Bluetooth speaker and battery-powered tea-lights was still a challenge in the sleepy half-dark of the delivery room. Playlist on and romantic lighting in place, she was ready for the big push. It had never struck me before quite how forcefully you have to push to get a baby out through your vagina. She was straining so hard it looked like something might burst that definitely shouldn't; I was alongside throughout trying to stay composed. Hand-holder, cheerleader and flannel dispenser, with the occasional semi-professional check of what was happening down at the business end. For half an hour or so it seemed like very little was happening, but soon, I could see the top of a head poking through the vaginal opening.

The soundtrack to this miracle of life unfolding before my eyes was the heartbeat of my child providing an almost gameshow-like timer sound effect from the CTG machine beside the bed, accompanied by the dulcet tones of Bruce Springsteen blaring through the Bluetooth speakers. The wonderful midwives were slightly worried by the occasional slowing of the heart rate and were contemplating involving the doctors to help the final few pushes with an instrumental delivery. They had one last trick up their sleeve to try first to get this baby out without any further delay. Out came the local anaesthetic and the episiotomy scissors. If you'd told me this would happen a week earlier, the thought would have sent shivers down my spine, but to even an untrained eye it would have been obvious that this head wasn't coming out without a bit of help. A gentle reminder from the midwives that a small controlled cut would prevent significant tearing and it was done. Seconds later and there it was, the head of my daughter, admittedly covered in the gunk of labour, but out and pretty normal looking. With one more push, the shoulders and body followed. She was a little blue at first but after what felt like an eternity, though was in reality only a few seconds, that all-important first cry broke the silence.

I'd always had the greatest respect for my wife, but looking at her lying on the bed with our new baby in her arms as I stepped forward to cut the gristly umbilical cord, I was truly in awe at the amazing physical and psychological battle she had just won - all carried out with the greatest decorum, strength and humour a partner could ever have hoped for.

What Women Want

DO come equipped with sweets, an ice pack and bucket loads of encouragement and compliments.

DO ask the midwife or obstetrician if you need clarifications or have any concerns.

DON'T let your fear show. Control your emotions and provide calm reassurance at all times even if that's not how you're feeling on the inside.

12

Baby

The first sweaty hours of dad life

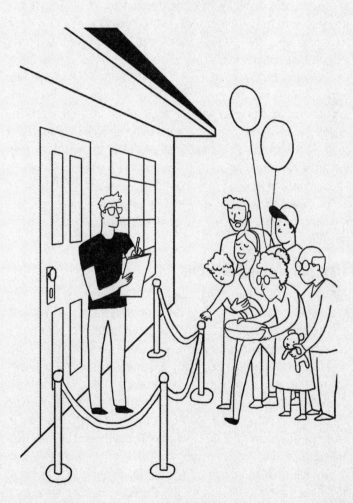

FROM THE DOCTOR

Finally, after what may have seemed an eternity, you are now a dad: congratulations! As soon as the baby is born, the team will carry out a very brief Apgar score test assessing heart rate, breathing, colour and responsiveness, to ensure that all is well and no additional support is required. This Apgar score is recorded at one and five minutes after birth, normally so subtly that neither you nor your partner will notice it happening. It's your new child's first exam. Most babies will be healthy on delivery, but sometimes it's necessary to give them some extra medical support. In these circumstances, the paediatricians will be involved and may initially take baby over to a special trolley, known as a resuscitaire, which looks a bit like a buffet hotplate. The trolley is equipped with oxygen and breathing tubes to help with respiratory problems and medications to treat early signs of infection. If there are any ongoing issues, your baby may need to be taken by the specialist team to the special care baby unit (SCBU) or occasionally to an intensive care unit. At every stage, the team will explain what's happening and why any intervention is necessary. Sometimes action needs to be taken very quickly to support baby, so try to remain calm and rest assured that all will be explained as soon as possible.

First parenting decisions

Within minutes of becoming a dad, you'll find yourself embroiled in parenting decisions. One of the first will be whether you and your partner would like your child to receive a dose of vitamin K – essential for blood clotting, this vitamin is present in very low doses at birth. Giving a new baby a top-up of vitamin K prevents against the rare, but potentially dangerous, disorder, haemorrhagic disease of the newborn (HDN). It can either be given as a single injection into baby's thigh within 24 hours of birth, or orally in separate doses over the first month of life. Although immediately inflicting an injection upon your new baby might seem harsh, in reality it's nothing compared to the head-squishing trauma of birth that they've just been through. Expect a cry, but after a quick cuddle and feed all will be forgotten. If you can't face it, then the oral drops are a good backup option, but ensuring the baby takes them can be challenging and subsequent doses may get forgotten in the chaos of the first month of parenting – so there's a risk baby may not receive the full course.

If your baby's birth was an uncomplicated vaginal delivery, it may be possible for your new family to head home within hours of the birth, as long as the midwives and doctors are happy. If a baby is born in hospital, on average, first-time mums spend a day and a half on a post-natal ward after a vaginal birth. If your partner had a C-section, she may stay in for an extra day or two, but many units are now encouraging women to go home earlier than this if they're recovering well.

There are post-birth assessments for mum and baby

Whether you're in hospital or at home, within the first 72 hours, a specialist midwife, doctor or paediatrician will perform a top-to-toe examination of your new arrival. They will be checking your baby for any signs of disease or disorder and assessing that all the necessary reflexes are working. A hearing test is normally performed before you leave hospital to screen for hearing problems. If not done in hospital, or you've had a home birth, this should be arranged within the first month by your midwife or health visitor. Total or partial hearing loss can significantly affect a child's development if it's not identified, so early testing is vital. A small, soft-tipped ear piece (like a tiny headphone) is inserted into the baby's ear and a series of clicking sounds are played. Sometimes, if baby won't stay still or there's some fluid in the ear from the birth, the initial test doesn't work and a second one will be required. You'll be given the results immediately and if any hearing loss is identified, an appointment will be made for your baby to be seen in the specialist audiology clinic for further investigation.

If your partner's been in hospital to have her baby, the health-care team will have a checklist of things to tick off before they're happy to discharge her. First up is the post-delivery wee. They will want to be sure that your partner is able to pass urine without any problem, particularly if she's had an epidural or a catheter in place. Don't be surprised if they actually ask to see the evidence – she may be given a cardboard bowl to pee into, so they can satisfy themselves that the waterworks are in operation once more. They will also want to examine your partner's abdomen to ensure that the uterus is contracting and take some basic observations to eliminate signs of infection, such as a fever or racing pulse. If your partner had a C-section, the scar will be checked to ensure there's no early signs of infection and the midwife or nurse will want to make sure that your partner can safely walk to the bathroom before she's let loose. Good pain relief and keeping the bowel movements regular will help to speed up recovery. The chance of deep vein thrombosis is particularly high after pregnancy and surgery, so the team may also recommend some blood-thinning medication to take home if your partner's risk is thought to be high. Finally, they'll want to be sure that you're happy with however you're planning to feed baby, whether breast or bottle, as feeding issues, leading to dehydration, are one of the most common reasons for babies and their mums to be re-admitted following birth. Now's the time to ask the midwives for help as they've seen and done it all thousands of times before.

Now you're home as a family

Eventually, whether it's hours later or after several excruciating days of watching your baby recover on the special care baby unit (SCBU), the time will come for you all to go home. There's no driving licence or qualification required to take your new baby home, but there's one thing that you will need before anyone will let you go anywhere – unless of course you live close enough to walk – and that's a car seat! Babies must be in a secured car seat at all times when travelling by car and for newborns this should be rear-facing, and ideally strapped or clipped into one of the back seats. If using a rear-facing car seat in the front passenger seat, the front airbag must be disabled (see Chapter 9 for more on this).

Whether you're driving your new family home, being driven by somebody else or taking a taxi, practise fitting the car seat before the big day arrives. Working out exactly which bit the seatbelt clips into or how the seat connects to its base is 100 times more difficult when it's loaded with precious cargo, you're suffering from lack of sleep and trying to look after a partner who has just given birth all at the same time. Time spent tinkering in advance will save a huge amount of gadget-related dad stress on the day.

Arriving home can bring with it a huge sense of relief – finally you're at one with your new family and away from the hustle and bustle of a busy hospital or clinic. But it might also be the time that you begin to wish that there was a parenting qualification you could have taken, as you suddenly realize you're flying solo – but of course, you aren't. There will always be friends, family and a team of midwives, health visitors and doctors to help you all along the way, and the next few chapters will give you some top tips for getting through those first six weeks of new-parent life.

Whether you're admiring the slowly deflating birthing pool in the corner of the kitchen or helping your partner to cut off her hospital name tags, taking it easy over the next few weeks is the key to success. Having a baby, no matter which method finally did the trick, is an exhausting process for mum, both physically and mentally. Needless to say, you'll probably be feeling it a bit too – perhaps more mentally than physically – but with some exhaustion thrown in for good measure. No matter how keen you are to show your new baby to the world, don't over-plan anything. Friends and family will be desperate to visit, so think carefully about when and how you release the news that you've arrived home. No matter how close the visitors, entertaining in any capacity is exhausting in the days after birth, so keep all visits short.

As the dad, managing the visitors is going to be one of your key roles – you're essentially the dad equivalent of a nightclub bouncer, just hopefully without the need to check the ID of the guests. Your first job is to remind people politely (in advance) that yes, you'd love to see them, but probably not for more than 45 minutes. The best visitors will do something to help, for example, bring a meal you can heat up later, unload the dishwasher or hold the baby while your partner has a shower. Even better ones will bring a bottle of wine to go with the meal and clean the whole house for you, but not all friends can be that amazing.

Your first few days will seem like a series of passing milestones. The first time you put your baby down to sleep, the first time they feed without help and, often the most feared by women – her first post-baby poo. The thought of squeezing out a first poo, particularly if she has had stitches or a tear, can be terrifying. Luckily, the thought is far worse than the reality. Pooing is not going to worsen the situation down below or tear things further, but some simple steps can make this understandably scary hurdle more manageable. If you're not in the business of discussing this sort of 'business' with your partner by now, this may have to change – support here is very important. Don't let her hold it in due to fear. After birth, many women don't open their bowel for the first day or two, but holding things in for longer because they're worried about doing more damage can lead to constipation and far worse problems down the line. Encourage her to poo gently when the time comes. Tell her not to strain too much, just allow the bowel to do its business. When she's sitting on the toilet, give her a small foot stool, or a pile of books or toilet rolls, to raise her feet so that her knees are above the level of her hips. This will line things up into the optimum poo-passing position. If constipation is a real issue, or there's been a particularly severe tear, ask the midwife or your doctor for some laxatives to use in the short term. Keeping well hydrated and eating plenty of fresh fruit and vegetables as well as wholegrains will help too. Reassuringly, most women report that their first poo wasn't nearly as bad as they'd thought it would be.

Some vaginal bleeding after birth (called lochia) is normal, whether your partner had a vaginal delivery or a C-section, as the uterus sheds its lining. Most of the bleeding comes from the site where the placenta was attached to the uterine wall and it can last anything from two to six weeks. It starts as heavier, brighter-red bleeding, which settles after a few days, and by the end of week one there will be smaller amounts of darker-coloured blood. Tampons shouldn't be used in the first six weeks after birth as there's a risk of infection. So, expect your partner to be using some pretty heavy-duty maternity pads, particularly in the first few days – think more incontinence pad than slimline, low-profile period pad. Breastfeeding stimulates the release of hormones that encourage the uterus to contract, so it's normal for your partner to feel some mild period-like cramps during breastfeeding and she may even notice that lochia increases when she feeds. Changing pads regularly and avoiding lots of lochia sitting near to the healing vagina will reduce the risk of any tears becoming infected. If bleeding becomes very heavy or your partner is passing lots of clots or is beginning to feel unwell, this could be a sign of abnormal bleeding, known as post-partum haemorrhage (PPH). If you're at all concerned, contact your midwife or doctor immediately for advice.

You'll be pleased to know that you really aren't alone

Your partner will have been given a contact number for your healthcare team so you can get in touch with them for advice at any point in the first couple of weeks. A community midwife will normally visit at home or make contact on the first day and either continue to visit for the next few days or arrange for your partner and baby to come to see the team at a local clinic. At every visit the midwife will check in to see how you're all coping. They'll ask how the feeding is going and examine your partner to make sure that the uterus is continuing to contract and that there are no signs of infection at tears or C-section scars. They'll want to check over the baby and after a few days will weigh them as this is an important guide as to how well they're progressing and feeding. You'll be asked how many wet and dirty nappies you've been changing, too.

When your baby is 5 days old a midwife will perform a newborn blood spot screening, known as the heel-prick, or Guthrie, test. This test checks for a number of rare, but potentially serious, medical conditions such as sickle-cell disease, cystic fibrosis, hypothyroidism and a number of other metabolic disorders, which, if detected early, can be appropriately treated or supported. Most babies will be unaffected, but the benefits of early detection are huge. Your midwife will make a tiny prick with a needle in your baby's heel and squeeze four spots of blood on to a special card. It really isn't very painful, but the holding still and squeezing usually isn't popular with babies, so be prepared for some crying. The results will either be sent to you by letter or given to you by your doctor or health visitor by the time your baby is 6 weeks old.

Midwife visits will continue up until your baby is about ten days old, and may go on for longer if there are any difficulties or complications. Around day ten, your local health visitor will conduct a 'new birth' visit and come to meet your partner and baby for the first time. Health visitors specialize in supporting mums and babies in the first years of life and will be able to provide endless advice and information on feeding, changing, soothing and caring for your new arrival – and your partner. After the initial home visit, your partner will be directed to the health visitor's drop-in 'baby clinics' where they'll keep a careful eye on your baby's weight as well as giving your partner the opportunity to ask questions or get support with her new life as a mum.

The famous red book

Shortly after birth, you will be given a personal child health record for your baby, commonly known as 'the red book'. This is a log book for all your child's health details, from the time of birth onwards, and is available in both paper and digital formats. It should be taken to all appointments with midwives, health visitors and doctors. As well as loads of other important details, your baby's height, weight and head circumference will be plotted on growth charts that enable the healthcare team to track your child's development over time. The red book also has loads of useful information for parents about child development, telling you what you might expect your child to be able to do, and when these new-found skills might kick in. It's well worth a read.

There are legal aspects to take into consideration

While you're in paperwork mode, registering your child's birth is a legal requirement. All births in England, Wales and Northern Ireland need to be registered before the child is 42 days old (in Scotland it must be done before 21 days), and there is often a bit of a wait to get an appointment so booking early is vital to avoid missing the deadline. Registration will normally take place in the Register Office local to where your child was born. Be sure to check what information and identification documents you need to take to the appointment and don't forget to take the 'red book' as many registrars will want to see this. Heterosexual couples who were married at the time of birth or conception can have both parents' names recorded on the birth certificate even if only one parent attends. If parents are unmarried, both names can only appear on the certificate if they attend the registration together or a specialist declaration of parentage form is completed in advance. Rules differ slightly for both male and female same-sex couples, so be sure to check all the requirements before attending your appointment.

If you're planning to jet off abroad with your new baby, whether on a world tour or simply to meet the family, they will also need a passport, and no birth certificate means no passport. Once you have the birth certificate, you can get the passport form to start the ball rolling. This also comes with the challenge of getting your baby to pose for some mugshots (without you in the photo), and don't forget that passports can take several weeks to arrive; even the fast-track service takes up to a week. So, whatever happens, don't book international travel before you have the passport in your hand. Different airlines have different regulations about flying with a newborn baby, with some permitting travel once they're two days old and others not allowing them on board until they're at least two weeks. You may also need a letter from your doctor confirming that your baby is safe to fly, so check with your airline well in advance of any planned travel.

FROM THE DAD

After an hour or so of cuddling and having her first breastfeed, the midwife asked me to bring my daughter over to the scales to be weighed and given her vitamin K injection. This was it, this was the first time I would hold her in my arms. I think all dads-to-be wonder what that moment will feel like and the media all too often tells of the instant love and adoration you'll feel as soon as you set eyes on your newborn child. I, like most of the dads I've spoken to, think this is overhyped. My overwhelming emotion was relief that both my wife and daughter had come through birth safely. I was entranced by the tiny bundle of towel-clad human that I carried across the room like a priceless ancient vase and I felt extremely protective, but the love grew with time. So, don't worry if you're not smitten beyond all belief within minutes; in fact, I'd say one of the greatest joys of becoming a dad has been the way in which my love for my daughter has grown on an almost daily basis, and indeed continues to do so.

As we headed to the post-natal ward, with its thermostat set to Sahara mode, the full exhaustion of the last sleep-deprived couple of days finally kicked in. There was just time for a brief rest before the midwives had me on what felt like a daddy-day-care boot camp. My advice is to make the most of having the experts so close at hand. I learned some excellent nappy-changing and dressing tips, which took me, within minutes, from a fumbling novice terrified of breaking a tiny arm as I forced it into a sleep suit, to a semi-pro ninja changer who is no longer defeated by poppers, no matter how many apparently hidden fastenings the designer has deceitfully concealed.

I'll never forget the night we spent in hospital. I was given a reclining chair to sleep in next to my new little family. But the mechanism was somewhat sensitive, so when I reclined, as long as I remained completely still, then there I would stay. A single twitch, however, and I was abruptly thrust back into a sitting position in an ejector-seat fashion with an almighty crash loud enough to wake all the babies within earshot. In the end it didn't really matter, because as soon as the staff turned the lights down for the night, my daughter decided that this was her moment to properly greet the world and she wouldn't stop crying. There were two problems with this. First was my wife, who was beyond exhausted and clearly needed to sleep if she was going to be able to function at all. Secondly, all the other inhabitants of our ward bay, who, although presumably equally exhausted, had babies that were seemingly quite on board with the whole day-night routine already. The dad-shame prevailed and I spent the night with my daughter in my arms pacing up and down the ward, making small talk with the midwives and sitting in the day-room. If this opportunity for further sleep deprivation had been on a list of optional extras at check-in, I would certainly not have selected it. But as I sat gazing down at my firstborn, desperately trying not to fall asleep myself, I was hit with the realization that this miniature human was entirely dependent on me and that this would be just the first of many pivotal bonding moments in our relationship - the love was kicking in.

Although the staff were fantastic, we couldn't wait to get out of hospital and start our new life at home together. Finally, all the checks were over, the precious cargo was loaded into her car seat dressed in a very oversized onesie, and we were off. Parents talk about arriving home with their new baby and suddenly wondering what on earth they should do next. I can honestly say we never felt that way. Arriving home felt so good, not just because I could finally escape the furnace-like temperatures of the post-natal ward, but because our daughter was finally part of our life, in our home, amongst our things. No matter how imperfect, we were now a family unit and I felt pretty sure she'd let us know exactly what she needed us to do next.

What Women Want

DO take the lead on nappy-changing while your partner gets to grips with feeding and recovers from birth.

DON'T let visitors in too soon and when they do come, don't let them stay for too long. Everyone will get very tired very quickly.

Feeding

Nipples, latching and milk machines

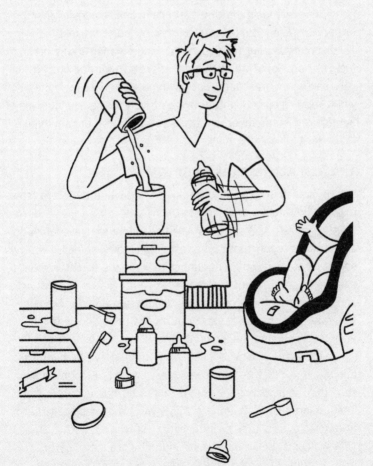

FROM THE DOCTOR

We all need food to survive and newborn babies are no exception. Though, in fact, they need very little in the first 24 hours after the birth as they have significant energy stores left from their time in the uterus. Feeding can cause a lot of stress for couples in the first days of parenting. Your partner may feel as though she's failing if she's struggling to establish breastfeeding and you'll probably feel like a fairly unhelpful bystander – without the ability to lactate through your own nipples. In fact, a well-informed and supportive dad can make a huge difference to her in the early days. Blame nobody – everyone's learning – stay calm and remember that the priority is to keep your baby fed and nourished. Which method your partner ends up using will depend on a combination of support and luck. There's a lot of pressure, applied by both men and women, for your partner to breastfeed, but for some women it simply doesn't work. Topping up with bottles or exclusively formula feeding may be required – remember that breast may be best, but anything is far better than nothing at all.

The first attempts at feeding

During that first hour of your baby's life outside the uterus the midwives will help your partner to try breastfeeding if she wants to. Plenty of skin-to-skin contact will help with bonding and doubles up as the perfect opportunity for an attempt at the first feed. If you've seen videos of newborns bobbing their heads across a mum's chest and seeking out the nipple (a reflex known as rooting), you'll know that there's a natural instinct to search for the boob. In reality though, few babies perform like the videos and lots of encouragement may be required.

Encouraging a baby to 'latch' on to the nipple can be difficult and opinions differ as to the best way to do this. Start by making sure that your partner is comfortable and has everything she needs nearby. Breastfeeding is thirsty work and keeping hydrated is important, so a large glass of water within easy reach is always very welcome. While both mum and baby are learning this new skill, a couple of pillows on the lap or a breastfeeding cushion to position the baby nearer the breast can help. Lying your baby on their side, 'tummy-to-tummy' with mum and with their head next to the breast, is a good starting position too.

A good latch is important as it minimizes trauma to the nipple and reduces the chances of your partner suffering from chapped nipples or developing infections like mastitis in the breast. When baby opens their mouth and they're brought towards the breast, they should raise their head and indent the breast with their chin first. It's not just the nipple that needs to go into a baby's mouth, they should take a large mouthful of areola (the darker breast tissue surrounding the nipple), too, and the nipple should be directed towards the roof of the mouth. If a baby is feeding well, you'll see the jaw muscles moving and be able to see them swallowing milk. If they're sucking in their cheeks or making a lot of noise, they're probably not latched on correctly. Breastfeeding may feel strange or uncomfortable at first, but if it's painful, encourage your partner to insert her little finger into the baby's mouth to break the contact and try latching the baby on again.

Things normally get easier with practice and staying calm is the key to success. For women who want to breastfeed but are struggling, there will be support available locally. Speak to your midwife or health visitor, as they have a wealth of experience in supporting women getting to grips with breastfeeding. They can also give you details of local support groups, where experienced breastfeeding advisors help those who are new to the challenge. Some babies are born with a tongue-tie, where the skin connecting the tongue to the floor of the mouth is shorter than normal. For many babies this won't cause any problems, but for some it may make feeding more difficult, so if in doubt ask a member of the healthcare team to check your babies tongue. If the tongue-tie is affecting feeding then they can be referred to a specialist clinic to have the tie cut – a painless procedure that takes seconds.

Your partner may also feel self-conscious about feeding in front of strangers or even friends and family. In a culture where women mainly cover their nipples, getting them out in front of your father-in-law or other family members can take some getting used to. Although there's nothing to be ashamed or embarrassed about, help your partner to feel comfortable when she feeds. Find her a private space or give her a shawl or muslin to cover herself with while her confidence grows.

Same nipple, different milks

During the first 2–3 days of your baby's life, your partner will produce a highly concentrated, nutrient-rich, milk-like fluid known as colostrum – which may have been leaking out of the nipples in the run-up to birth. Colostrum is so rich, and baby's stomach is so small, that they only need about a teaspoon (5ml) at each feed – less than a sip of milk for an adult mouth. If your baby is struggling to latch on or is a reluctant feeder for whatever reason, your partner's midwife may help to hand-express the colostrum into a feeding syringe. This involves gently squeezing the breast and 'milking' the colostrum towards the nipple, where it can be collected, drop by drop, into a syringe. This can then be fed directly into the baby's mouth, so you know they're getting food in the early days.

After 3–4 days your partner's milk will start to 'come in'. The arrival of this 'mature' milk is normally announced by the sudden swelling or engorgement of the breasts. By now your baby will probably be more awake and be ready for a feed, too. Breast-milk production works on a supply-and-demand basis – the more your baby feeds, the more milk your partner will produce. If in the first few weeks she feels she's not 'making' enough milk to meet the demands of a growth spurt, reassure her that by feeding more regularly, if necessary, the supply will increase as your baby stimulates production. Sucking on the nipple also stimulates a 'let-down' reflex, so that as the baby latches on, milk stored within the breast is pushed down tiny ducts until it reaches the exit at the nipple. This reflex can be pretty powerful, so don't be surprised to see milk squirting from your partner's nipples while she is helping the baby into position. Just hearing a baby cry, or thinking about feeding, can be enough to trigger this reflex. Likewise, feeding from one breast can cause milk to squirt from the other. While a supportive feeding bra will help to keep breasts comfortable, nipple pads, disposable or washable, are vital to prevent the leaking of milk through clothes and keep the nipples dry.

It's not always plain-sailing

If feeding isn't going well, nipples and breasts can start to get pretty sore. Nipple creams are also useful to prevent sore and cracked skin that is not only painful but also a route of entry for bacteria and possible infection. Women who produce a lot of milk can also develop engorged breasts, which are sometimes so full that it's difficult for the baby to latch onto the nipple. Ask the midwife or health visitor to show your partner how to hand-express or use a breast pump to release a little milk, which may make it easier for the hungry milk-guzzler to latch on. Don't overdo the expressing though or the breasts will just produce even more milk, thinking they're compensating for a hungry baby – it's all a balancing act.

Each breast is divided into segments – imagine the sections of an orange – and tubes, or ducts, drain milk from the segments towards the nipple. Sometimes a duct can become blocked, causing a firm painful swelling in the breast. Usually the key to freeing this is to encourage your partner to continue feeding from the affected breast as this will help to unblock it. A warm flannel placed over the breast can work wonders, as can having a hot shower while gently massaging the breast. If your partner's breast is very painful, red and hot or she's feeling unwell or developing a fever, this may be a sign of an infection within the duct and breast, known as mastitis. In this situation a visit to the doctor is required as your partner is likely to need some antibiotics as well as pain relief. She'll also need some serious encouragement from you to continue feeding to get things going.

Breast is undoubtedly best

With all the potential for stress, chapped nipples and milky bras, you may be thinking why bother breastfeeding at all? Well, breast-feeding provides a huge number of benefits to both baby and mum and it's recommended until the baby is 6 months old and weaned on to 'solid' foods – but you can breastfeed for longer. The majority of women start by breastfeeding, but as the weeks pass, many give up for a host of different reasons. The good news is that even a short period of breastfeeding will bring benefit to your baby, but the protection and benefits increase the longer it's continued.

Breastmilk is a perfectly designed cocktail bringing nutrition and health benefits that are far greater than those offered by formula milk. Mum's immunity is passed to your baby, which reduces the risk of infections, but research shows it also reduces the risk of cancers, such as leukaemia, sudden infant death syndrome, cardiovascular disease and obesity to name just a few. The hormone production breastfeeding triggers also offers protection to mum that is often overlooked. Women who breastfeed also have a reduced risk of developing breast and ovarian cancer, cardiovascular disease, obesity and osteoporosis (thin bones). There are practical benefits too. Most importantly, breastmilk is free and readily available at the right temperature, wherever your partner is, saving time, money and the hassle of all the bottle-feeding paraphernalia like bottles, teats and sterilizers. Expressing milk and giving it from a bottle is a great way to reap the health benefits of breast milk while giving your partner a break and also means you get to have a go at feeding too. Expressing can be done by hand or by using a breast pump. Pumps are far more efficient and come as either manual or electric models. A suction funnel sits over the nipple to stimulate milk release and it's all collected in a little bottle that can then be fed to your baby. Expressed breastmilk in a sterilized container can be stored in the fridge (at 4°C/39°F or lower) for up to 5 days, the ice compartment of a fridge for up to 2 weeks or the freezer for up to 6 months. If your partner is breastfeeding, avoid trying to introduce milk in a bottle for the first few weeks, or until feeding is well established. The process of feeding from a bottle is very different from latching onto a nipple and confusion can occur if things are made too complicated. There's a balance to be struck though; if you want to introduce a bottle, don't wait too long either as you may find that your baby decides that breast really is best and simply won't feed from any other source.

Feeding equipment must be sterilized

Whether expressing breastmilk or giving your baby formula milk, you'll need to get to grips with the sterilization process as this may well come into the dad list of responsibilities. It's recommended that you sterilize all feeding equipment for the first 12 months of baby's life to reduce the risk of infective illnesses from bacteria, viruses and parasites. The first step is to wash all the equipment (bottles, teats and caps) thoroughly in hot, soapy water. You can use a dishwasher for the cleaning phase, but it doesn't sterilize, so there's still work to be done. There are three common ways to sterilize baby feeding equipment: using a steam sterilizer, cold-water sterilizing or boiling the kit in a pan of water. Steam sterilizing is popular as it's the most hassle-free. You can buy relatively cheap sterilizing boxes or bags that can be filled with feeding equipment, topped up with a bit of water, and put in the microwave for a few minutes, or invest in a more expensive free-standing steam sterilizer. Whichever method you choose, follow the manufacturer's instructions carefully.

Cold-water sterilizing uses liquids or tablets that are dissolved in water in a lidded container designed for the purpose. Check the manufacturer's guidelines to see how much water should be added to the chemical and be sure to change the solution every 24 hours. Submerge all of the feeding equipment making sure there are no air bubbles in bottles and teats and leave for at least 30 minutes. Once they've been sterilized, you'll need to rinse the equipment with cooled, boiled water before filling them for the baby.

The cheapest way to sterilize is to simply boil the feeding equipment in a big pan for at least 10 minutes; ensure everything remains below the surface so it gets the full sterilization effect. Check that any equipment you're planning to plunge into your cauldron is safe to be boiled. But be aware, too, that teats and bottles may not last as long if being boiled regularly.

Making up formula milk

If you're using formula milk in your proudly sterilized bottle, you'll also need to learn how to prepare it. Formula milks are usually cow's-milk-based products, so check with your midwife, health visitor or doctor that you're using the right product for your baby. You can buy pre-mixed milks, which can be poured straight into your freshly sterilized bottle (great if you are away from home), or for a more cost-effective solution, milks come in tins of dried powder that are added to water as and when you need to make up a feed – it's very important to follow the manufacturer's mixing advice precisely as formula powder isn't sterile. Boil the water to kill any organisms it might contain, pour the required amount into a sterilized bottle and leave it to cool for up to half an hour, allowing the water to reach 70°C/158°F. Then add the powdered formula – don't put the powder into the bottle first. Put the teat and lid on the bottle and shake to make sure it's thoroughly mixed. Bottled mineral water isn't sterilized, it just comes fresh from a mountain stream somewhere, so isn't free of infection risk and shouldn't be used. Finally, before you offer your baby the freshly prepared bottle, make sure the milk is at an appropriate temperature that won't burn baby's delicate palate. Test a few drops of milk on the inside of your wrist to check the temperature before starting a feed – it should be warm but not hot. You can cool a bottle by holding it under a cold running tap. If you need to warm a bottle, whether formula or breastmilk, submerge the bottle in a bowl or jug of hot water until it reaches the desired temperature. You should never use a microwave as these can cause pockets of scalding milk that may burn your baby.

The dad bottle time

When giving a bottle, make sure that both you and your baby are comfortable. It's important to maintain eye contact to offer reassurance during the feed. Hold your baby in a slightly upright position, supporting the head and neck. Allow them to touch the bottle and become familiar with it. Sometimes squeezing a drop of milk onto the teat is helpful, so they get a first taste without too much effort. Most importantly, always make sure the teat is full of milk otherwise the baby will be gulping down large mouthfuls of air along with the tasty stuff, which can lead to trapped wind and may come back to haunt you later.

After the feed, support your baby in an upright position to help bring up any air they may have swallowed. Either do this on your lap, supporting the head and neck with one hand and gently rubbing or patting the back with the other one, or pop them against one of your shoulders and gently pat or massage the back.

So just how much milk does a newborn baby need?

Stomachs start off very small, about the size of a small marble, so fill and empty very quickly. In the first week or two it's unlikely your baby will be in any fixed feeding pattern; some days they'll want to be fed every 1-2 hours but on others they'll go as long as 4 hours between feeds. Every baby is different, so be guided by yours, but don't let a new baby go more than 4 hours without a feed, as at this stage there's a risk of the blood sugar becoming too low, which kick-starts a cycle of sleepiness and even less desire to feed. Aiming for at least 8 feeds a day is a good rule of thumb. For breastfeeding and bottle-feeding new mums, the best strategy is what's known as responsive feeding. Feed either because baby is giving feeding cues (sucking fingers or fists, rooting or wriggling towards the breast) is crying, or if your partner's breasts are becoming uncomfortable, engorged and need to be emptied. This 'responsive' feeding technique aims to respond to the needs of both mum and baby - don't worry, it's virtually impossible to overfeed a breastfed baby.

If you're formula feeding, your baby will probably be needing feeds of 30-90ml in the first week, increasing to 75-105ml by weeks two or three. If you fancy a bit of maths, from week two onwards most full-term babies need 150-200ml per kg of body weight in a 24-hour period. So, work out the total, divide by the number of feeds per day and you'll get an idea of how much the little guzzler should be taking on board at each feed. Don't let your partner panic about getting into any kind of feeding routine too soon. Most babies take about 12 weeks to establish a regular feeding routine (and some never do). Remember that night-time feeding is important too as this is when the body produces most prolactin - the hormone responsible for triggering breastmilk supply. So, feeding at night helps to boost the milk supply. Sorry, I know that's not the news you wanted!

FROM THE DAD

I think my daughter had her first breastfeed within the first hour of being born, thanks to a little help from the midwife. After all the talk of the special moment, it got rather lost in everything else that was going on and the general excitement of the new arrival. Unfortunately, that was the easiest feed she'd have for the next 24 hours. Despite regular midwife encouragement and my wife's perseverance, this baby was not interested in nipples or milk. All she wanted was a bit of sleep and perpetual cuddles. We weren't particularly concerned, safe in the knowledge that she'd have enough reserve to get her through the first day without extra food. This relaxed approach suddenly disappeared when we discovered we wouldn't be discharged home until she'd safely established feeding.

No amount of nose-to-nipple, shaping and shoving or natural breast-seeking instinct seemed to be working, so I encouragingly stood by as the midwife helped my wife to 'milk' her own breasts and express the colostrum into a tiny syringe - sucking milk drop by drop from a self-squeezed nipple is easier said than done and not a very rewarding task. What felt like hours of effort finally resulted in the most miniature of milkshakes that didn't look big enough to sustain a few cells, never mind a screaming baby. Expressed milk should be handled like priceless liquid gold because a simple slip or spill will almost certainly result in tears from your partner and the most incredible feelings of guilt that you've ever experienced - spill any form of breastmilk at your peril, you have been warned.

My turn soon came

Having aimed to be a hands-on dad, not being able to directly share in the feeding - as my partner had chosen to breastfeed - made me feel a bit redundant. I seemed to be missing out on this amazing bonding experience. But I did find solace in becoming the self-appointed chief water boy and cushion adjuster until we introduced a bottle of expressed milk at around 4 weeks. An amazing warmth surged through me when I looked down at my own child gulping down every-thing she needed from the breastmilk 'smoothie' that I'd so lovingly prepared. Once you've started the bottle, never stop (I repeat, never stop) and keep up the practice at least twice a week. I made the mistake of stopping for a month or so, and by the time I brought the bottle back, my daughter's love for it had totally vanished. Hours of screaming followed any attempt to encourage her to even put the teat in her mouth and any onlooker, or listener for that matter, would have thought there was a baby torturer in the room rather than a doting dad trying to feed his hungry child. This girl knew what she wanted and, for several weeks, the bottle was certainly not it.

The baby weigh-in

Throughout the first few weeks, your midwife, then the health visitor will be weighing your baby. Like boxing pre-match weigh-ins, the stakes feel high. As new parents enduring sleepless nights of latching, feeding and sterilizing, any weight loss feels like a public shaming of your meticulous training regime.

Weight loss is to be expected in the first week of life; many babies lose 7-10 per cent of their birthweight. Don't panic though, most will have regained their original weight by 10-14 days if all's going well with feeding. Any figure or target is a danger for a new dad, especially me. I realized I was becoming overly fixated when I reached for the kitchen scales, changed the nappy and tried to do some 'home weighing'. Not only is trying to keep a newborn baby safely balanced on small kitchen scales more challenging than getting a good grip on a wet bar of soap at the bottom of the bath, but a daily weight competition does nothing for team morale. So, my advice is to leave baby weighing to the pros and use your scales as they were intended and bake a cake for your partner instead.

What Women Want

DO set up comfy areas for feeding, complete with plenty of water, snacks, the TV remote, chat and encouragement (this is particularly important for night feeds and especially in the first week).

DON'T suggest that every time the baby cries it's because your partner hasn't fed them enough, even if this could be true.

Crying

Why is everyone at it?

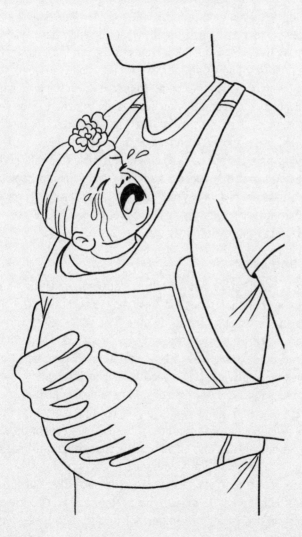

FROM THE DOCTOR

For months you've been waiting to hear your baby's very first cry – you may even have had to wait a few nervous seconds longer once they came into the world. But now you're probably beginning to wish they'd stop. Crying can be one of the biggest challenges for new parents, causing significant psychological stress. Unfortunately, crying is your baby's only real way of making their needs known to you and, like all communication, it will take a few weeks before you and your partner are able to identify what's behind a particular cry.

Nature has been vaguely kind to us though, as most babies cry less in the first 24 hours after birth than they do in the weeks that follow. Being born, whether being squeezed down the birth canal or delivered by C-section, is an exhausting experience for your baby too, so much so that they are likely to cry a lot less for the first day. So, make the most of it and rest as much as possible. From then on, crying may increase week by week, with babies typically crying for 3-5 hours each day. There are a few perfectly healthy babies at it for up to 12 hours a day – yes, that's right, half the day. The good news is that crying typically peaks at around 6 weeks of age and things tend to improve after that.

Why babies cry

Crying is your baby's way of letting you know that they need something, but sadly, they can't yet tell you what. In the first couple of weeks, it's safe to assume that your baby is crying because they are hungry. In the early days most aren't particularly bothered by dirty nappies, but as the stomach is so small and so quick to empty, offering a feed is a good first option. Some breastfed babies cry almost constantly until the mature, free-flowing breastmilk 'comes in' (see Chapter 13 for more on this). This is probably because the breast hasn't quite caught up with what the baby needs and is still only producing colostrum. Rest assured that continuing to feed regularly will encourage the milk to come in and your baby will soon settle once their nutritional needs are being met. If you or your partner are ever concerned about excessive crying, it's important to discuss this with your midwife, health visitor or doctor to make sure that there's no underlying physical cause – most of the time, luckily, there won't be.

Stopping the crying

Attending to your unsettled baby quickly in the early days and weeks is felt to reduce the amount of crying long-term, so prepare to respond and comfort them quickly. Of course, this isn't always possible to do safely if you're having a shower or driving the car at the time, but evidence suggests that as long as the majority of crying is responded to sympathetically, the occasional prolonged bout will not do any harm. Remember, no matter how hard it might be in the middle of a sleep-deprived night, your baby isn't crying to annoy you, it's just all they know how to do. If a cuddle or a feed doesn't settle things, there are a number of other tricks to have up your sleeve.

After months of being in your partner's uterus your baby will have become accustomed to the sound of her heartbeat and of blood 'whooshing' through the vessels. Recreating this in any way you can will often help, so embrace the opportunity for skin-to-skin cuddles before cuddling Dad is the last thing they want to do. Baby-wearing, using a sling or harness, is also worth a try as it creates a warm, reassuring environment that's close to the sound of your heartbeat. Babies who are carried or 'worn' regularly often cry less than those who aren't. Gentle repetitive sounds that are similar to the sounds of living inside a uterus may also soothe your baby. The noises made by a dishwasher, vacuum cleaner or washing machine are often the secret to soothing success. If you don't fancy constantly running your domestic appliances or just don't like vacuuming, many parents swear by a 'white-noise' track – you can download these to your smart phone or tablet. If sound isn't the answer, try movements like gentle rocking or swaying. Taking your baby out in the car or for a walk in the buggy or in a sling may also help them settle if things are getting really desperate. Finally, don't overlook the power of the 'bum pat'. Holding your baby in your arms, use one hand to gently and rhythmically pat their bottom. This is said to simulate the reassurance of a heartbeat and is used by midwives on post-natal wards across the country. They should know!

As the weeks pass, you'll start to understand why your baby is becoming distressed. Hunger remains a common cause, but now your baby may cry if they are uncomfortable after a feed, scared by a loud noise, unwell, have a dirty nappy, have experienced emotional distress, or have developed colic or reflux (more on that to come). Don't panic about not being able to identify these immediately; it comes with time and all new parents get there eventually – soon it will just seem obvious.

Wind, possets and the dreaded colic

A common time for babies to become unsettled is during or immediately after a feed. Burping is a skill that both you and your partner will soon become masters of. Whether breast- or bottle-fed, babies will often develop trapped wind during feeds and being able to quickly relieve this for them will save a lot of tears. In reality, gravity is your saviour here. You need to get your baby in an upright position, so gravity can pull the milk downwards, allowing the bubbles of air to float to the top and come up out of the foodpipe (oesophagus) as one big burp. The easiest way is to sit baby on your lap, supporting the head and neck with one hand and using the other to press gently into the lower back to straighten the spine. Either rub or gently pat the back and before you know it, the burp will be with you. Alternatively hold the baby against one of your shoulders and again, gently pat or massage the back until you hear that all-important sound. Never before will the sound of a burp have brought so much joy to your life.

If you've ever held a baby, and the proud parent has kindly covered your shoulder with a muslin square first, you'll probably be aware of the risk of a little milky regurgitation from time to time, also known as a 'posset' – milk, mixed with stomach acid, that comes up the oesophagus and out of the mouth. The ring of muscle that acts as a valve between the top of the stomach and the oesophagus takes months to fully develop, so it's very normal for milk to escape and for babies to posset several times a day. The acid-infused milk coming up the food pipe can be pretty uncomfortable for the baby – if you've ever suffered from indigestion, you'll know the feeling. Feeding in a more upright position and keeping your baby upright for 20–30 minutes after a feed will really help.

While most babies cope well with occasional posseting, some will have more severe symptoms known as reflux, or to give it its full name, gastro-oesophageal reflux disease (GORD). Symptoms include prolonged crying after feeding, back-arching and irritability. If your baby is growing well and putting on weight, it's likely that they'll grow out of it by the age of one when the muscular valve at the top of the stomach is fully developed. But if your baby is really suffering, not putting on weight or vomiting more severely, you should contact your health visitor and/or doctor for advice. Once they've identified the cause as reflux, baby-safe antacid medications can be used to help settle the symptoms.

Most babies cry more in the early evening and nobody knows for certain why, although it's thought this might be because milk production is at its lowest at this time of day. However, if your baby is crying for long periods every night, they may be suffering from infantile colic. It affects about one in five babies worldwide – it's seen equally in both boys and girls and breast- and bottle-fed babies. Typically, it is periods of crying, fussing or irritability lasting at least 3 hours a day, at least 3 days a week for at least 1 week. Babies may clench their fists and/or draw their knees up to their tummy or arch their backs when crying. Some experts argue that this may just be part of the normal spectrum of baby crying while others hypothesize about different gut bacteria or abnormal gut movement and pain signalling being the cause.

The key thing as far as a parent is concerned is that your child will be otherwise healthy, growing well and thriving – despite the crying. The good news is that most babies grow out of colic by 3–4 months, but if your child suffers badly, it can make the first few months of parenting a particular challenge. Remember a few things: first, that it isn't either your or your partner's fault – your baby will grow out of it – and, secondly, looking after the mental well-being of both your partner and yourself is vital so that you can adequately care for your child during this difficult time. Techniques to help improve things include all of the soothing techniques described, as well as trying warm baths, gentle tummy massage and moving baby's legs in a cycling motion in an attempt to release any trapped wind.

You can buy over-the-counter colic remedies at pharmacies and even supermarkets. Some parents find they make a big difference and others find they don't help at all. They are thought to help by gathering all the smaller air bubbles together to form larger bubbles that can more easily be released out of one end or the other. Some remedies can be used from birth – but others including old-fashioned gripe water shouldn't be tried until your child is at least 1 month old. Check with the pharmacist. The old-style gripe water (no longer available), contained some alcohol, but needless to say giving alcohol to your baby to get them to stop crying – no matter how tempting – is bad parenting and not allowed. Sorry!

The dummy debate

Some parents choose to use a dummy, or pacifier, to help soothe their baby. If your partner is breastfeeding it's advisable not to introduce a dummy until your baby is 4–6 weeks old, or until breastfeeding is well established. Sucking on something else can not only confuse a baby but it also makes it more difficult for you to know when a feed is being demanded. Whatever you do, don't listen to the grandparent classic advice of dipping the dummy in sweet treats like honey – unless you want a baby with rotten teeth. If you and your partner have decided to try a dummy, go for the 'flat teat', or orthodontic, dummy as these seem to be least likely to damage tooth development. Make sure you give your baby plenty of 'dummy free time' so they can get to grips with babbling and start to develop the early stages of speech. There's some evidence that sucking on a dummy can increase the risk of middle ear infections, but other research suggests that using a dummy at night might reduce the risk of sudden infant death syndrome (SIDS), also known as 'cot death' – debate is still ongoing in both of these areas. But if crying is becoming your nemesis, a bit of dummy action, even just for a few months, might be your saviour.

Parenting a crying baby can be an emotional rollercoaster

A baby that cries a lot can make the early months very challenging for parents. Finding ways for both you and your partner to cope with this is very important. Give each other time away from the baby so you can both have some time to yourself, without the crying soundtrack ringing in your ears day in day out. If you've got friends or family who are willing to do a shift, even just an hour or two away can really help both of you. Sometimes people reach breaking point and feel so frustrated with a crying baby that they become tempted to shake them or start having other negative thoughts towards their baby. If either you or your partner feels this way, the safest strategy is to put your baby in a safe place, such as the cot, close the door of the room and leave them to cry while you take some time to re-group or get some support. You can always call your health visitor.

If by now you haven't given up the whole idea of having a baby or have started to look into giving up your new arrival for adoption, it may horrify you to discover that it probably won't just be baby tears you'll have on your hands. Becoming a parent is undoubtedly a very emotional experience. Combine this with a painful front-bottom, sore nipples and sleep deprivation and this can soon turn into an emotional tear-fest. Hormonal changes are thought to be responsible for the very common 'baby blues' that your partner may experience in the first week after birth. These feelings of upset, anxiety and sometimes just, 'What on earth have we done?' are completely normal and affect more than 50 per cent of all new mums, and should settle by about 10 days after birth. As a new dad, you may be experiencing a similar emotional rollercoaster, but trying to be available to support and reassure your partner is vital. Remembering that the experience is very normal will help and, if you can, use a bit of humour to try to turn the tears of desperation into tears of laughter instead.

Post-natal depression can affect both parents

If symptoms of low mood, tearfulness or difficulty bonding with the baby continue beyond two weeks, your partner or you may be suffering from post-natal depression. This can develop any time within the first year of birth. It affects at least one in ten mums and is increasingly being recognized in dads, too. The emotional and physical changes of becoming a parent as well as the change in relationship dynamics can all have a huge effect on mental health. Sadly, these feelings can become so severe that parents may begin to have negative thoughts about their baby. It's important to identify symptoms of post-natal depression as soon as possible and to remember that it's almost as likely to affect you as it is your partner. Many new parents find it much easier to talk to their health-care team about the physical difficulties of parenting than the psychological ones, but your midwife and health visitor are there to help. They will regularly check on the mental health of both parents in the weeks following birth. Hospitals have specific teams responsible for looking after mental health in the perinatal period and early intervention with talking therapy or even antidepressant medication can prevent symptoms becoming severe or a crisis point being reached.

The most severe, but luckily by far the most rare, mental-health condition that can affect women in the weeks after birth is post-partum psychosis. Hallucinations, thoughts or beliefs that are unlikely to be true, manic behaviour or paranoia may all be symptoms. Women with this condition often don't realize they're unwell and if you think your partner is developing the symptoms this should be treated as a medical emergency, to prevent her causing harm to either herself or the baby. As with all post-natal mental-health conditions, it can affect women with a history of mental-health problems or strike for the first time in somebody with none, so if you're concerned, get medical help straight away.

FROM THE DAD

I was prepared for my daughter to cry and even expected my wife to be tearful, but what took me by surprise was the ease with which the tears would suddenly start flowing. In the first week, I'd often come into the room to find my other half truly sobbing - previously a very rare occurrence. Luckily, these seemed to be mainly tears of joy as she was bowled over by the intense love she felt towards our new arrival. I felt almost guilty; was I a bad parent for not feeling the same way? Perhaps my bond was taking longer to form. The health visitor, maybe insensitively, asked at her first home visit when my wife was planning to go back to work. The result: more tears. Other dads have told me they found themselves mopping up tears in the middle of department stores simply because a bra or Babygro wasn't available in the right size. One reported a full meltdown when a bunch of flowers brought by a kind visitor started to die. My advice is to prepare to gently support but don't feel the need to rationalize or explore every emotional outburst.

Becoming a dad is undoubtedly an emotional challenge; whether you're a bawler, just shed the occasional tear or you're so hardcore you've never cried in your life, things may be about to change. Post-natal mental health issues in dads have been poorly recognized for many years, but luckily this is changing. Having a baby can have an instant impact on your relationship with your partner, financial security, free time and social network. As if sent as a sinister reminder, about two days before my daughter was born, a young dad came to see me in my clinic with a story that really made me reflect on how I was going to cope emotionally with having a child. He was worried that he wasn't bonding with his six-month-old daughter. He had a busy job and every time he came home, he had to spend time caring for his daughter and wasn't able to spend any of the quality time he'd previously enjoyed with his wife. He was exhausted, felt incredibly low, was now performing badly at work and had started to have suicidal thoughts. He was clear that he loved his wife and wanted to feel the same way towards his daughter, but his life had been so de-railed by her arrival that he couldn't see a way through. The guilt surrounding his feelings was palpable and when I told him I thought that, like nearly one in ten dads, he was suffering from post-natal depression, he looked shocked. Instead of him struggling through with the assumption that he was simply morally corrupt, or in some way unloving, I reassured him that he had not only a recognized, but also a very treatable condition. He asked me as he left if I thought he'd be able to love his daughter as he so desperately wanted to. I was confident that with the right treatment he would and the visible look of relief that came across his face as he digested the news will remain with me forever. Do not underestimate the power of changing circumstances to affect your mental health, no matter how hard, manly or stoic you may think - or wish others to think - you really are.

What Women Want

DO master some good soothing techniques so you can take over once your baby is fed and your partner is exhausted.

DON'T mention anything to do with hormones when your partner is tearful in the first weeks. Just gently reassure, comfort her and give her a big cuddle.

Pooing

Getting down and dirty beneath the nappy

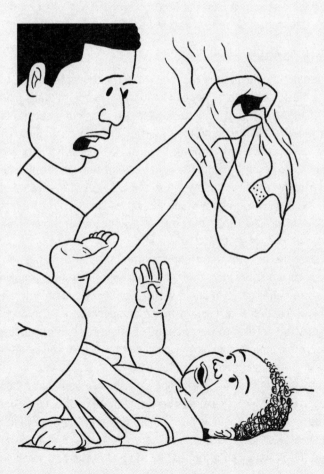

FROM THE DOCTOR

It's often said that having a new baby is just a cycle of eat, poo, sleep, repeat, and it can certainly feel like that in the first few weeks. The baby sleeps and you may or may not be helping with the feeding, but the nappy-changing is one task that invariably falls to dads. Even if you can't do anything else you can wipe up the shit. Or can you? If you haven't changed a nappy before, knowing what's normal and the best way to do it often causes concern for new parents. A top tip is to ask the midwife to help you the first time you step up to the mark. Then embrace all of the advice available from experienced parents, too.

Dirty nappies

Your baby should do their first poo within 24 hours after birth, but it's a black, sticky, tarry deposit known as meconium that's made up of all the digested amniotic fluid, mucus and other substances that they've swallowed on their journey through pregnancy. This first bowel movement is notoriously sticky and difficult to wipe away, so go gently but persevere. As dads so often get the pleasure of changing the first nappy, the sticky, wipe-resistant meconium can seem like somebody's set you up as the victim of a very successful practical joke, but you're not alone. Generations of men and women have struggled before you.

Over the next three or four days the meconium changes to a green-brown substance, then gradually gives way to a yellower, mustard-coloured semi-liquid with a weirdly sweet smell if your baby is breastfed. Like mustard, the grainy appearance is completely normal and nothing to worry about. Formula-fed babies will have a more toothpaste-like, pale-yellow or brown textured poo that smells more like the real deal adult variety.

If you didn't have ninja nappy skills before your baby came along, fear not. Practice makes perfect and you're on a nappy boot camp – what will begin as a 15-minute fiasco at the beginning of the week will soon be a slick military operation. Your baby will need a new nappy so often that by the end of the first week you may have done it more than 100 times. In the first week, some babies poo after every feed but expect around 4 dirty nappies each day on average. By the second and third week, you may notice things start to settle down, although some babies will continue to open their bowels after each feed, while others begin to go without for longer periods. Your baby may not open their bowel every day. This is completely normal as long as they're comfortable. It's also normal for a baby to strain and go red when they're opening their bowels. But if they're uncomfortable or passing hard, pellet-like stools this may be a sign that they're suffering from constipation. If you're worried, discuss this with your doctor or health visitor. Other warning signs to look out for include chalky, pale-white poo, which might indicate a blockage in the liver, or fresh blood in the stool. If you spot either of these call your doctor as soon as possible.

Wet nappies

Hopefully there will be plenty of peeing going on too. Passing urine is a good sign that your baby is hydrated and feeding well. You don't have to change the nappy every time your baby does a wee, but in the first week, you should aim to change it at least every 3 hours, and always if there's poo involved. Urine should be light in colour and not offensive-smelling. Dark, smelly urine can be a sign of dehydration or infection. Modern nappies are so absorbent that they soak up most of the urine and you'll start judging how much has been produced based on how heavy the nappy feels. As a guide, during the first week or two, 8 wet nappies a day would be completely normal, with fewer than 6 being a warning sign that dehydration might be occurring.

If you've had a girl, in the first week you may notice a small amount of white vaginal discharge, which is sometimes a little bloodstained. This is completely normal and just the result of the withdrawal of mum's hormones that she's been exposed to in the uterus. Don't worry, this will be her last 'period' for many years and should settle on its own.

Which nappies?

So now you know what's going into the nappies – which type will you choose, disposable or reusable (cloth) nappies? Buying disposable nappies can become expensive so reusable ones might offer a more cost-effective and environmentally friendly solution – as long as you have a low-energy washing machine and aren't tempted to tumble-dry. In an attempt to reduce nappies being put into landfill, some councils offer vouchers towards buying reusable nappies. Before you start panicking at the thought of the constant washing, it's possible to buy biodegradable, disposable nappy liners to use with reusable nappies. Supermarkets and pharmacies are filled with different disposable-nappy options, some of which are also biodegradable. Some disposable nappies come with added features like having a line on the front that changes colour to let you know when your baby has wet themselves, but sadly, none seem to have developed a good poo detector – yet. Some people go for a combination, choosing reusable nappies most of the time and using disposables when they're out and about.

The changing bag

Whether you go eco-friendly reusable or hassle-free disposable, you'll need to get a nappy bag packed to take with you to the hospital. From that day onwards, failing to restock any of the key ingredients will bring potential disaster to any day out. Every good bag needs:

NAPPIES OF CHOICE   In the first week, a nappy for every hour or two you plan to be away from home.

CLEANING EQUIPMENT   Either baby wipes or cotton wool and a pot of water for cleaning up after the inevitable. Baby wipes should be suitable for newborns and alcohol-free. Water-only wipes are a convenient alternative, if more expensive.

NAPPY BAGS   Keep enough to dispose of the offending nappy and to stash away any clothes that get caught in the cross-fire.

CHANGING MAT A fold-up travelling changing mat will be vital when you end up changing your baby on the floor or even the so-called 'clean' baby-changing surface of a motorway service station. Always best to have your own mat and not rely on the cleanliness of others.

BARRIER CREAM A tube of your chosen barrier cream for if things start to get a bit red and sore down below.

CHANGE OF CLOTHES You will need to have at least one clean set of clothes – that's for the baby, hopefully not you too.

How to change a nappy

You've got all the gear, so now how do you change a nappy without getting everything everywhere – at home or when you're out and about? Here goes:

GATHER UP EVERYTHING YOU NEED IN ADVANCE Make sure the new nappy and cleaning stuff, and change of clothes, if needed, are all within reach. Taking your eye off the ball for just a second to search in a bag or drawer after the nappy is off can result in a faecal fiasco that you'll regret for hours as you attempt to half-wrestle half-dance your way back into control. If you fail to prepare, prepare to fail.

CHOOSE A SAFE PLACE Ideally lie your baby on their back on a changing mat or towel. Changing tables are great, but the floor is by far the safest. Never leave any baby unattended on a changing table. Even though newborn babies can't roll over, as babies grow they wriggle and roll with increasing skill, which puts them in imminent danger if they're left unattended at a height.

UNDO THE NAPPY Hold both your baby's feet in one hand and lift upwards to keep them out of the way. Try to maintain eye contact with your baby, reassuring them and smiling; don't give them the dirty look that their nappy might deserve – although in reality baby poo is mostly pretty inoffensive.

CLEAN YOUR BABY'S BOTTOM Use the dirty nappy to wipe away the worst of the poo and then use either cotton wool and warmed water or alcohol-free baby wipes for the detailed clean. Wipe all of the skin within the nappy area, paying particular attention to the skin creases as it's easy to miss bits.

FOR GIRLS Wipe from front to back, in an attempt to prevent bacteria from the poo entering the vagina or urethra (pee hole) that may increase the chance of urine infections.

FOR BOYS Wipe the testicles and the penis, but there's no need to clean behind the foreskin.

ROLL UP THE DIRTY NAPPY Use the tabs to seal it shut before putting it into a nappy sack. Disposables can go in an outdoor bin. Reusables can be put in a nappy bag or bucket, ready for washing later. They need to be washed at 60°C and it won't be long before you have a machine-load's worth ready.

PUT ON A NEW NAPPY Slide the new nappy under your baby's bottom; typically the sticky tabs go at the back and attach at the front. Make sure the nappy is pulled high enough up, well beyond the buttocks into the small of the back. Bring up the front between the baby's legs and pull the tabs firmly around to stick on to the front panel. Check that the nappy is firmly closed and that the frilly bits around the thighs are pulled out to prevent leakages.

WASH YOUR HANDS Always wash your hands afterwards to prevent passing infection to your baby.

A word of warning: young babies have little or no control over their bowels and bladder, so be aware that whenever the nappy is off, more poo or pee could come your way. If there's a penis involved, the hose-pipe effect may mean your face and eyes are in danger of a drenching, so always remove a nappy with caution. Some people put the opened-out, clean nappy underneath their baby before removing the old one, so that it's in place as soon as the dirty one is off. This avoids the few seconds of nappy-cross-over danger, where both you and the mat are fair game for soiling.

Nappies and the cord stump

If you cast your mind back to the birth, you'll remember the umbilical cord being cut and clamped. One of the plastic clamps remains on what's left of the cord, until the 'stump' dries and eventually falls off (sometime between one and two weeks later), leaving a newly formed belly-button. While the stump dries it's important to keep it away from the contents of a dirty nappy. Until the belly-button is formed, always fold the front of the nappy down so that the stump remains above it. Many newborn-sized nappies have a 'cut-out' at the front to protect the stump. Once the stump's fallen off, there will be a small wound at the belly-button site for around 10 days until it dries out. It's normal for this to look a little mucky and sometimes even bleed a little on to clothes or nappies. If the area is becoming very red, it smells offensive or your baby is becoming unwell, contact your midwife or doctor.

What causes nappy rash?

When the bacteria in the stools combine with the urine inside a nappy, they produce a substance called ammonia that can be very irritating to a baby's skin and can cause nappy rash – red inflamed skin around the nappy area. Some babies' skin will be more sensitive than others, but the key to avoiding nappy rash is regular nappy-changing. A wet nappy is less of a problem but try to change dirty nappies as soon as possible. Applying a thin layer of barrier cream on babies with sensitive skin or at the first signs of redness gives the skin some protection between changes. Nappy-free time is important too. Lie your baby on a changing mat in a warm room with a clean, new nappy underneath them. Allowing the skin to air-dry and giving it time without direct nappy contact can quickly help any nappy rash to heal. If the skin is starting to get red, antiseptic creams can be used regularly to help settle symptoms and for more severe outbreaks titanium-based creams are very helpful. If the rash persists, contact your doctor or health visitor for advice.

FROM THE DAD

Years before I'd even thought about having a child, I'd occasionally see a parent making a mad dash for the baby-change facilities carrying, at arm's-length, a child with a dirty nappy overflowing right up its back. This was a disaster that I'd always attributed to bad parenting, rubbish nappies or a baby with a serious bowel problem. Worse, I'd mistakenly assumed that the 'poo-nami' would never be a problem that would cross my parenting path. How wrong I was. I was happily marvelling at how unfussed my daughter was by sitting in her own faeces when I realized that her latest release was not just confined to my perfectly sealed nappy, but had in fact travelled all the way up her back, covering the car seat and everything else in its path in a sweet-smelling, highly staining, yellow poo-dye that required high-strength stain remover to return any fabric to even a close resemblance of its original colour. The poo-nami is not simply the preserve of the incompetent parent. A well-fitting, well-fastened nappy can help minimize the risk, but a combination of liquid faeces, the baby's position and the explosive nature of a new baby's poo means they're a constant hazard. In the aftermath, consider carefully just how special the soiled outfit really is and whether or not your darling child is about to outgrow it anyway - sometimes throwing out the worst-affected item and cutting your losses is the best strategy. Failing that, buy an extra-large pack of the best stain remover you can lay your hands on (suitable for sensitive skin) and prepare a sink or bucket for a good scrub-and-soak session.

The risk of being peed on by a baby was something I was more familiar with in my life as a doctor. Learning to avoid having a baby piss in your face as you remove the nappy to examine them is up there with the top survival tips for any doctor starting out in paediatrics. Boys' penises are well known for doing the 'hose-pipe' trick, perfectly aiming a powerful 'water' jet into the onlooker's eye, but it's the girls you have to watch out for. These wees are far more covert, often unnoticed by the nappy-changer fixated on tabs and frills, until they try to do up the sleep suit only to discover the back is completely soaked. Cue a full outfit change and, despite my best fashion intentions, rarely, if ever, does my choice meet with my wife's approval unless strict guidelines have previously been issued.

Poo-namis away from home

Resolving the collateral damage from a poo-nami is hard enough on home turf, when you'll have a well set-up changing station and ample kitchen towel and nappy bags to hand. But changing on the fly is a whole different game. My heartfelt thanks go out to all those public venues that provide clean, spacious nappy-changing facilities for parents in the midst of a nappy nightmare, particularly those who have finally understood that a dad may be stepping up to the task, where hiding the baby changing area in the ladies' loos is just not OK. The sight of a man with a poo-covered shirt, carrying a baby, poking his head around the door of the ladies' toilets is humiliating for both parties. That said, armed with a portable changing mat, I've become adept at what I like to call extreme changing. I have found that anywhere from the relatively controlled confines of the back seat of a car to the grassy kerb of a motorway have been fair game in an emergency. The floors of gents' toilets are less desirable though; for the first time in my life I, too, have learned to hate men who sprinkle when they tinkle.

What Women Want

DO get handy at nappy changing and know how to pack the changing bag for trips out of the house.

DON'T be surprised when poo goes all up your baby's back, or when your partner suggests you should clean it up.

Sleeping

That'll be the baby, not you!

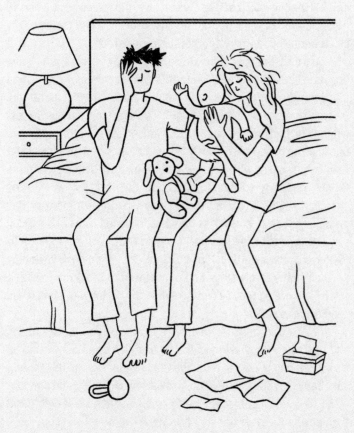

FROM THE DOCTOR

You may have turned to this chapter rather nervously, afraid of discovering what you already know in your heart to be true. Any friend without a baby will delight in reminding you that as a new father, your sleep pattern will, undoubtedly, be disrupted. In nature's clever way though, you've probably been on a slow sleep-deprivation training programme for the last 40 weeks with your partner getting up all night to go to the toilet or tossing and turning with the discomfort of a heavy pregnancy bump. What you may not know is that newborn babies sleep a lot – most sleep as much as 18 hours in any 24-hour period. It's just that they don't necessarily sleep when you fancy getting some shut-eye too.

You'll find that your baby will be very sleepy on day one as being born is exhausting. Yet again, nature is on your side, as this gives you and your partner the chance to recover from the birth marathon. Be sure to make the most of this. Encourage your partner to rest when your baby sleeps, and get as much rest in as you can, too, because the peace will not last. The bad news is that after this brief respite, newborns will normally only sleep for 1–3 hours at a time, waking regularly to demand food. In the first few weeks, the circadian rhythms that let them know whether it's night or day aren't developed, so as far as they're concerned 2am is a perfectly sensible time to have a lunchtime snack. The best strategy is not to fight it: a pattern will develop with time. On a more positive note, a newborn baby rarely stays awake for more than 90 minutes at a stretch, so even if they're crying constantly during that time, it will soon come to an end.

In those precious first weeks, be guided by your baby's needs and ride the rollercoaster, grabbing as much sleep as you can as it's too soon to try to get them into any routine. By the third week, your baby may start to develop an awareness of night and day, and by 6 weeks, most babies will be sleeping much more at night time than during the day. You see, I promised some relief. From week three, it's worth helping your baby to learn to distinguish between day and night. During the day, keep things light and bright, engage in eye contact and play with your baby. At night, particularly during feeds, keep the lighting low and avoid eye contact or overstimulation. This may seem unfriendly at first, but your baby will be reassured by you and your partner's presence, and parents who've had at least some sleep tend to be in a much better frame of mind to care for their child.

If you or your partner were hoping for a few early nights in the first weeks then think again. Newborns are often awake (and crying) in the evenings and demand lots of feeds. Many won't settle until around 11pm and that's after a cluster of evening feeds, so you may find your new arrival joining in on dinner and box-set plans rather more than you would have liked. The concept of bedtime is unlikely to appear until a baby's about 8 weeks old, when a few start sleeping through the night. Each baby is different and there are no set rules, so don't beat yourselves up if someone else's baby is sleeping 'better' (or just a bit longer) than yours. They may just be experiencing the calm before the storm. Avoiding the temptation to compare is a valuable parenting self-care skill.

You'll soon become an expert at soothing your baby. Try not to get into any ridiculous habits like driving them around the block every night to get them to sleep, or you may end up doing this for months to come. There are lots of different soothing techniques in Chapter 14, and you'll soon find something that works for you and your baby. It's also a great opportunity to bond with your baby and there's little better than the satisfaction of successfully getting them to fall asleep in your arms.

The art of swaddling a baby

This ancient practice of wrapping a baby in a muslin or thin blanket has been used for centuries to help very young babies fall asleep. It comforts the baby as it mimics the sensation in the uterus and prevents them waking themselves by jolting their arms and legs and, if done correctly, it's actually been shown to reduce the chance of cot death. The art falls somewhere between wrapping a present and folding a fajita wrap, where your newborn child is the sizzling mixture of peppers and spicy flavourings. Follow one of the many online 'how-to-swaddle' videos for your first attempt and you'll be a master in no time.

Parents worry about sleeping babies

It's often said that there is nothing more peaceful than a sleeping baby. This is true, but unfortunately there's often nothing less peaceful than parents watching over a sleeping baby checking to see if they're breathing. A baby's breathing can be very shallow, at times almost convincing onlookers that they're not breathing at all. Understandably a huge fear of new parents is cot death, or sudden infant death syndrome (SIDS). Fortunately, this is rare, with around 300 babies dying a year from SIDS in the UK. The exact cause is still unknown but is thought to relate to how babies regulate their heart rate, breathing or temperature in response to environmental stresses. Parents can easily let their worries become out of control, so the best policy is to follow advice from your midwife or health visitor, do all the things that we know reduce the risks and then just relax.

As young babies aren't good at regulating their own body temperature you can help by making sure they don't become too hot or cold. For many years babies were put to sleep on their front, but in the early 1990s the 'back-to-sleep, feet-to-foot' campaign was launched, which significantly reduced the number of cases of SIDS. So, what does this mean? First, lay your baby on their back to sleep so they are less likely to overheat or bury their face in the mattress; don't be tempted to put them to sleep on their side as they may roll onto their front. In addition, position them so that their feet are at the foot of the cot, pram or Moses basket; this way if a baby kicks and wriggles during their sleep they can only push themselves up away from blankets and covers rather than sliding underneath them and running the risk of overheating or being smothered.

The room where your baby sleeps should be 16-20°C/60-69°F. Cover the baby with lightweight bedding or put them in a specially designed baby sleep bag – these are available in different weights, or togs, for different weather conditions. Never use a duvet in a baby's cot. Cellular blankets, the waffle-like ones with small holes in them, are ideal as they're very breathable, but sleep bags are good too, although have a higher price tag attached. If you want to keep a careful eye on the baby's temperature there are loads of smartphone thermometer apps or specialist thermometers that can be plugged in near your baby's cot. Don't be over-focused on the numbers, but do keep a careful eye out for extreme temperatures such as searing summer heat or winter freezes. The best tip is to remember that your baby should wear one more layer than you need to keep yourself at a comfortable temperature. So, here's a rough guide as to what to dress them in.

Above 25°C/77°F: Vest only – baby's unlikely to need any blankets or sleep bags.

22–25°C/71–77°F: Vest and one layer of blanket or a 0.5–1-tog sleep bag.

18–21°C/64–70°F: Vest and a sleep suit with either a single layer of blanket or a 1-tog sleep bag.

15–17°C/59–63°F: Vest and a sleep suit with either two layers of blankets or a 2-tog sleep bag.

Below 15°C/59°F: Vest and a sleep suit with three layers of blanket or a 3–3.5-tog sleep bag.

What is the thinking on co-sleeping?

Your baby should sleep in the same room as you and/or your partner for at least the first 6 months. Babies who sleep in a separate room are almost twice as likely to die of cot death, but fortunately very few incidences of cot death occur after the age of 6 months. It's recommended that your baby should sleep in a cot or Moses basket in your room, but many mothers wish to sleep, at least some of the time, with their baby in their bed – known as co-sleeping. Debate rages about whether this is safe or not. Sleeping together can bring convenience and easy night feeding for breast-feeding mothers and can also help with bonding. Cot death is less common in breastfed babies, so parents of bottle-fed babies are advised not to co-sleep with their child. It's thought that breast-feeding mothers respond most safely to their babies while sleeping, so the guidance is that dads or other carers of even breastfed babies should not sleep alone with their baby in bed. Although mothers understandably worry about the risk of smothering their child, it's worth remembering that only 1 per cent of cot deaths are caused by accidental smothering in bed.

There are other reasons to avoid co-sleeping, too. Neither you nor your partner should co-sleep if your baby was born prematurely (less than 37 weeks' gestation) or with a low birth weight as there is already an increased risk of cot death in these groups. Neither you nor your partner should co-sleep if either of you smoke (even if not in the bedroom or the home), have been drinking alcohol or using drugs (this includes medications that may make you drowsy) or are suffering from extreme tiredness. Whatever happens, don't let yourself or your partner fall asleep with your baby on a sofa or armchair. With all the soft cushions, edges and crevices, doing this is associated with a significant increase in the chance of cot death.

If you're having nightmares about the risk of cot death, but want your baby near you both at night, a co-sleeping crib might be the answer to your problems. These are specially designed baby cots that attach to one side of your bed, with the nearest side folding down to allow easy access to your baby for those middle-of-the-night feeds. These bring all the convenience and closeness of co-sleeping without the risks and, importantly, leave all the space in the main bed for you and your partner. Nobody likes sharing that much when the precious commodity of sleep is at stake.

FROM THE DAD

Sleep deprivation is a recognized form of torture and whether you're an eight-hour fanatic or a born insomniac you're going to find your sleep pattern changing as soon as your baby arrives. Having done my fair share of night shifts over the years, I thought I'd be a natural. I had become pretty used to making important decisions at 4am or being woken from a brief sleep to attend a cardiac arrest, but the sleep deprivation that comes with being a new dad was somehow different. Whether it's night shifts, big nights out or a sleepless night ahead of an important meeting, periods of interrupted sleep normally have an end point, and are usually followed by the chance to have a lie-in or an early night to recover. Once I started life as a dad I quickly realized that there was going to be no day off, no rest day or real break from the sleep interruption - disturbed sleep was here to stay. But like with anything, I began to adjust, heading to bed a bit earlier when I could, happy in the knowledge that I'd probably be woken up several times each night.

The jaundice days

For the first few days, my daughter was incredibly sleepy, particularly at night time. A bonus you might think, but it turned out she was mildly jaundiced (more on this to come in Chapter 17). The result was that she slept more than usual, but it was important that she had regular feeds to keep her hydrated and flush the jaundice out of her system. Despite significant protest from my sleep-control centre we set an alarm to wake us up every 4 hours – if she hadn't already done so – to give her some more milk. On a few occasions, she was so sleepy we had to use some gentle encouragement, moving her around, taking off her clothes and even using a cool sponge on her bum to wake her from her slumber and get her latched on.

It's like sleeping in a farmyard

For light sleepers, nodding off next to a newborn can be a challenge. The noises my sleeping daughter made in the early days were so loud I could have been forgiven for thinking I was at a sleepover with a collection of farmyard animals. A constant rumble of snuffling, squawking and snoring filled the air, but it did at least reassure me that she was still breathing! She slept in a co-sleeping crib attached to the side of our bed, which was incredibly convenient for the night-time breastfeeding sessions, but – whether because of sleep deprivation or just new-parent anxiety – for the first few weeks I regularly woke up in a panic. I'd find myself fumbling around in the dark convinced that I'd either fallen asleep on top of her or that she was somehow missing from her crib. Inevitably, the panicked bleary-eyed search with the help of the light from my phone revealed that she was exactly where we'd left her and, unlike me, was sleeping soundly – well, farmyard soundly.

Sleeping strategies

For the first couple of weeks I'd get up with my wife when she was doing the night-time feeds to keep her company and give her some support while they both got the hang of breastfeeding. Once I headed back to work, being up all night wasn't ideal, so I'd try to do the early morning nappy-changing and entertainment shift before heading off for the day. Many dads I've spoken to have found different strategies to enable both them and their partners to maximize sleep. It all depends on who's doing what and when and whether people have to go to work, but there's likely to be a solution to at least ease the pain a little for you as a couple. Some dads simply slept in different rooms, others encouraged their partner to go to bed nice and early and gave the baby a bottle at around midnight before heading to bed themselves. That way their partners could have a good 6 hours or more of shut-eye before waking for the next breastfeed. Other couples came up with a combination of separated sleeping and role variation depending on the day of the week to fit in with work schedules and weekends off. It's worth trying a few options to see which works for you and if you try the midnight-bottle option, you'll find there's a perfect chunk of time each evening in which to write a book, with just a few minor interruptions from a hungry baby - I can vouch for that.

What Women Want

DO come up with a sleeping strategy that works for you as a couple, so you can both get as much rest as possible.

DON'T worry about other parents and how well they claim their children are sleeping; it's not a competition and they're probably exaggerating anyway!

Caring

Your baby under the bonnet

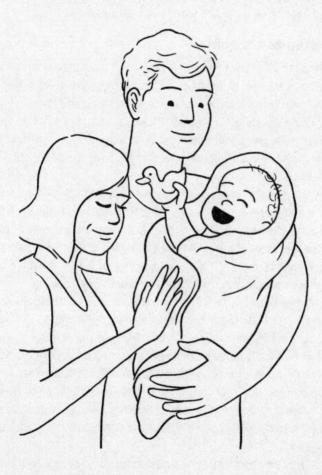

FROM THE DOCTOR

Most high-spec appliances you unbox at home come with a troubleshooting guide, but now you're probably gazing at your most precious delivery to date and wondering exactly what each button does and how it really works – under the bonnet. This chapter can't teach you everything, or I'd be writing a very long and rather boring paediatric textbook, but let's go top-to-toe as you lovingly survey your new baby and ask, is this normal? And what exactly are the maintenance instructions here?

The top-to-toe guide

After birth your new bundle of joy may well have a few bumps and bruises, particularly if they were born by instrumental delivery. These will normally settle over the first few weeks and shouldn't be any cause for concern. A paediatrician or specialist midwife will have already given your new arrival a structural once-over shortly after the birth, but if you spot anything you're concerned about, be sure to ask.

On top of the baby's head, you'll find a diamond-shaped soft patch and there will be another similar area towards the back of the head. These are known as 'fontanelles' and are simply areas where the bones of the skull have yet to fuse. It's perfectly safe to touch and clean them and they'll be present until the baby is at least one year old, when the bones will finally fuse together.

Birthmarks are incredibly common, particularly on the forehead, eyelids or neck. These can be pink or red v-shaped marks also known as 'stork marks' or 'salmon patches' that are present from birth and will normally fade and disappear within a few months. Other marks known as 'strawberry marks', or infantile haemangiomas, can appear in the first few days of life. These may continue to grow gradually for some time, but will normally resolve on their own. If they're particularly large or causing concern, ask your doctor to take a look.

Gazing into your baby's beautiful eyes, you may be wondering what they're seeing? The answer is that everything is pretty blurry to begin with. It will take about a year for your child to see the world as you do. For the first month they can only focus on objects 20-30cm away, just far enough to check out your beautiful facial features when you're holding them in your arms or wrinkling your nose at their dirty nappy, or to see your partner's face when they're breastfeeding. If you have particular hopes for your child's eye colour, don't get too excited too quickly. Many are born with blue eyes that will darken over the next 6-9 months; eye-colour is not normally established before the child is about one year old. Occasionally you might notice that one eye looks slightly inwards or outwards and the other one looks straight ahead. This is known as a squint. Occasional squint is very common in newborns and usually no cause for concern. It should have gone by the age of 3 months, so if it hasn't, or it's happening all the time – or if there is a family history of squints – talk to your health visitor or doctor.

About one in five newborns have either one or both of their tear ducts blocked at birth. This can cause watering eyes as the natural tear film has nowhere to drain and it can cause sticky or crusty deposits around the eyes after the baby's been sleeping. The ducts will normally unblock without help within the first year, but in the meantime, clean the eyes with cotton wool dipped in cooled, boiled water. Always wipe from the nose side outwards and use a separate swab for each eye.

Your baby may develop red or white spots on their face that look a bit like acne. That's probably exactly that what it is and 'baby acne' is very common. Okay, so it's not the most beautiful look for your social media feed in the early days, but if left well alone, the skin will settle on its own without any scarring. Don't be tempted to squeeze the spots as, just like in adult acne, it increases the risk of infection and of long-term skin damage, no matter how psychologically satisfying it may be. Rashes that don't disappear when pressed (most easily tested by pressing a clear glass onto the affected skin) could be a sign of serious conditions, such as meningitis, particularly if accompanied by a fever or your child appears unwell, and should be immediately reviewed by a doctor.

Is your baby looking a bit sun-kissed or like they've had a bad fake tan? Yellowing of the skin and whites of the eyes is a sign of jaundice, one of the most common conditions affecting newborns.

It can develop any time from the second day of life up to 2 weeks, but it's most likely to peak at around 2-3 days. It is caused by a natural process whereby red blood cells are broken down to form a yellowish substance called bilirubin, normally filtered out of the blood by the liver. In newborn babies the liver isn't mature enough to process the excess bilirubin and so it remains in the blood, causing the colour change. As long as your baby is well and feeding normally, jaundice will usually resolve within a few days and isn't normally a cause for concern. If you notice jaundice in the first 24 hours of your baby's life or it persists beyond two weeks, contact your doctor or health visitor. Normally the doctor will perform a blood test to check the level of jaundice and, if necessary, can treat it with phototherapy – a special 'sun-bed' lamp that breaks down the bilirubin into a form that the young liver can handle.

As babies' skin is exceptionally delicate, they're born covered in a layer of a whitish substance called vernix, which is their first fully natural moisturizer experience. Even though it looks a bit gross, try not to wash it off. Allowing it to soak naturally into the skin will help to nourish and protect the baby's skin as it adapts to life outside its uterine spa. Babies who are overdue will often have less vernix and may have very wrinkly skin, particularly on their hands and feet – a bit like when you spend too long soaking in the bath. This 'overcooked' look won't last long and you may notice some peeling of the skin on the hands and feet, revealing a fresh, soft layer of skin below.

Now to the maintenance instructions...

Tempting as it is to want to scrub and polish the new arrival like a gleaming trophy as soon as you get them home, they actually don't need a bath for their first week on planet Earth. For the first week, you and your partner can just 'top and tail' your baby, cleaning their face and the area underneath their nappy with warm water (ideally cooled, boiled water) and cotton wool. There's a lot of chat in baby books about cooled, boiled water and yes, it's as simple as it sounds. Boil water in a kettle, allow to cool to the desired temperature, check carefully that it's not too warm and then use this freshly 'home-purified' water to cleanse your child. Use separate pieces of cotton wool for the face, body and nappy area – and always a fresh swab for each eye. You don't need any soap or cream at this stage; just allow the natural vernix time to sink in.

After the first week, it's time to get baby bathing. Aim to bath them every 2–3 days, for short periods initially, until they get used to it. Some babies hate having a bath and new parents are always anxious about putting their little treasure into the tub for the first time. Try to hold back the nerves on the first few occasions as your baby will undoubtedly pick up on them and by the time you've done a week's worth, you'll be a confident washer-dad. You can either bath your baby in a special baby bath or in the main bath tub with a non-slip mat or baby bath seat attached to the bottom. Keep the bathroom warm, and check that the water is also warm – not even babies enjoy a tepid bath and nervous parents often make it too cool. Of course, it mustn't be too hot either. The skin on your elbow is particularly sensitive and a great place to check water temperature with, even if you do look a little weird elbowing the bath.

Once everything's prepped, and the towel is to hand, undress your baby down to their nappy. Wrap the baby in a towel and clean their face as if top and tailing, then hold them over the edge of the bath to rinse the hair and towel it dry. Lay the baby down again and remove the nappy, making sure they haven't done a cheeky poo while you've been elbowing the water and rinsing the hair. Obviously, if they have, this needs to be wiped away first – nobody wants a floater in their first bath. You'll be pleased to hear that babies almost never poo once they're in the bath, but a quick wee is fair game in the lovely warm water and not of concern. Gently lower them into the bath and if you don't have a baby bath or seat to support your child, put one hand around the upper back and hold the arm and support the head. Put your other hand under the lower back and bottom and lower the baby into the water. The first few attempts are best thought of as 'bath training' for both you and your baby, so keep them in just long enough for you both to get used to the idea. Newborns will become cold very quickly as they struggle to regulate their own body temperature, so a few minutes is all that's needed. Washing and holding at the same time is a higher-level skill that comes with practice. You can use the hand from the lower back to scoop water over the baby or, better still, another pair of hands can be very useful. Once you're both feeling more confident – which may take several baths for some babies (and their parents) – use a baby flannel or sponge to gently wash them, starting with the head and face and finishing with the bum and genitals. Not even a newborn wants their face washed with a cloth that's just been used on their bum. Key areas not to forget are behind the ears, folds of the neck and under the arms. Parents often bring babies in to see me with cheesy-smelling armpits and normally this is as a result of not getting into the crevices at bath time – you have been warned. Oh, and never leave your baby unattended in the bath.

Once the washing and fun is over, have the towel ready for a quick switch from warm bath water to cosy towel cuddle. Particularly in hard water areas, having a bath can dry out babies' skin, so you or your partner may wish to give them a post-bath massage with an oil recommended for newborns, to soften the skin and allow some bonding pamper-time after their bath. Be sure to get a nappy back on quickly to avoid having to repeat the whole washing process all over again.

Despite best bathing efforts, in the first few weeks you may notice some greasy yellow scaly patches that appear on your baby's head. Known as cradle cap, this is very common, it's not contagious, and it has nothing to do with bad parent bathing or hygiene skills. Cradle cap normally settles on its own within a few months, but if you want to speed things up you can use natural oils to soften the scales and wash your baby's head with a baby shampoo. Using a soft baby brush to gently brush their head after washing will help to loosen the scales, though may feel bizarre if there's no hair to speak of. Avoid the temptation to pick at the scales as this may break the skin and leave it open to infection. If you are concerned, talk to your health visitor.

A newborn baby's fingernails grow very quickly and cutting them can be a difficult job. Babies with long nails often end up scratching themselves and irritating the skin on the face and body, so keep them regularly trimmed. The challenge of a tiny target combined with a wriggling hand has led to many a parent coming to see me in tears having minorly cut their baby's finger. Some people say you can bite them yourself, but this is not recommended because it can introduce germs and leave jagged edges on baby's nails. In the first few weeks you can file the nails or cut them carefully with baby nail scissors or clippers, ideally when your baby is asleep, but be sure to keep the fleshy finger-pad out of the way. Be extra careful with nail clippers as they're very sharp and perfect for taking a chunk out of the wrong place if you don't watch what you're doing. Check the toe nails too but these usually don't grow quite as quickly as the fingernails.

Once they're washed, polished, trimmed and finally off to sleep, you'll no doubt continue gazing at your baby unable to believe that you were, at least half, responsible for bringing them into the world.

Symptoms to watch out for

There are a couple of things that newborns do that can be a bit alarming. The first is jerking. The occasional jolting movement, both when asleep and awake, is very normal as long as it only lasts for a second or two, and it will settle down as the nervous system becomes fully developed. Anything lasting longer than this requires urgent investigation. The second is irregular breathing. The centres in the brainstem that control our regular adult breathing take time to develop and so babies may breathe very shallowly and irregularly in the first 6 months of life, sometimes appearing to stop for up to 10 seconds, and this is quite normal. If, however, you notice a period where your baby stops breathing for 20 seconds or more before restarting, this may represent what's known as a brief resolved unexplained episode (BRUE) and you should call for an ambulance or take your child straight to hospital for review in a paediatric emergency department.

If your new baby develops a fever, becomes drowsy, isn't feeding as normal or is in any way causing you concern, call your doctor straight away and request an urgent appointment. Always remind the receptionist at the clinic of the age of your child and they should arrange for them to be seen quickly as young children can deteriorate very rapidly. If the clinic is unable to see your child and you're still worried, take them to the nearest emergency department for review. When a baby under the age of 3 months has a fever, don't give them paracetamol or ibuprofen unless advised to by a healthcare professional. They will require immediate assessment by a doctor to determine the cause of the fever before any treatment is started.

Post-birth check-ups for mum and baby

As the weeks fly by, you'll quickly feel more confident handling and caring for your baby and of course your health visitor and doctor are always available to answer any questions you may have. At 6 weeks, both your baby and partner will have a review appointment, normally with your doctor and health visitor. The doctor will arrange a double appointment, one for each of them, and this is another perfect opportunity to address any concerns your partner or you may have. Be sure to take along the child health record or 'red book' you were given as the doctor will perform another full physical examination of your baby, much like the one done shortly after birth. Your partner will be able to discuss any problems she's experiencing following birth and the doctor will check any healing wounds if she wishes.

Sex and contraception after birth

The six-week post-natal check is a good time for your partner to discuss contraception with her doctor – assuming, that is, that you don't want to enlarge the flock immediately. Even if your partner is breastfeeding and hasn't yet had a period, it's still possible to become pregnant if she has unprotected sex. Immediately after birth there's an increased risk of blood clots forming in your partner's veins so oestrogen-containing contraceptives like the combined pill, vaginal ring and patches are not recommended as they increase this risk further. Oestrogen may also cause difficulties with initiation of breastfeeding so it's advisable to avoid these for at least the first 6 weeks. If you're back in the game earlier than this, there are still plenty of options. The progestogen-only pill (or mini pill), contraceptive implant or injection, and male or female condoms can all be used immediately. Internal contraceptives –

the intrauterine device (IUD) and intrauterine system (IUS) – also known as coils, that sit in the uterus with threads coming through the cervix into the top of the vagina, can also be used. These can be inserted in the 48 hours immediately after birth or if the thought of that is too much to bear so soon, they can be fitted again from 4 weeks. Sex and pregnancy may be the last thing on both of your minds at this stage, but it's worth a little thought if you feel you could do with a few years' break before revisiting the pages of this book.

When is the right time to start having sex again? Well, there are no rules here, other than to say that you'll have to wait until both you, and even more importantly your partner, feel ready. Sleep deprivation, changing relationship dynamics, body image and even just the thought of having sex with your child nearby may have an impact on libido and are all feelings experienced by many of the dads I've met. When I bring up contraception at six-week checks with new mums, they invariably give me a disapprovingly knowing look. One woman summed it up perfectly: she looked me straight in the eye and, pointing to her vagina, said, 'Nobody is going anywhere near this for quite some time.' Don't forget all the other ways of being physically intimate without the need for penetration. When the time arrives use plenty of lubrication and take things gently – be guided by your partner, who'll undoubtedly be feeling nervous. Urinary leaking and incontinence following birth is experienced by some women, so support your partner to continue those squeezing pelvic floor exercises used during pregnancy and if symptoms persist encourage your partner to see her doctor.

Carving out time for you as a couple

This is always difficult in the first few weeks, but as things begin to settle, it's important to keep up whatever it is that makes you tick as a duo. A couple of hours away if somebody can babysit or even a meal out together with your baby sleeping in the buggy alongside can really help to hit the reset button. You'll be surprised how portable babies are in the first few months, so you shouldn't have to miss out on many social events once you start getting used to parenting life – unless you fancy using the baby as an excuse.

Hopefully by the time you and your family reach the six-week mark, you'll be finding your stride and more importantly your smile. It's around now that you can expect all of those dirty nappies, sleepless nights and hours of tortured crying to pale into insignificance as your baby finally smiles back at you for the very first time. Unhelpful onlookers will tell you 'it's just wind'. Don't believe them.

FROM THE DAD

I wanted to finish this book at the six-week mark not because there's no more science to understand or advice to give, but because I believe that from this point onwards, no other man, woman or book can tell you how it is that you should be parenting your child. There are countless guides that will advise you on sleep regimes, weaning, child development and behaviour if you so wish, but I feel passionately that the beauty of fatherhood lies in the unique approach that each dad will take to raising his children.

I hope that this book provides you with a guide to landing your new arrival safely on the planet and will help you keep them fed, happy and clean for the first few weeks. But - critical as this is - it represents only a tiny fraction of your life as a dad and of your child's existence in the world. We learn parenting skills from our own parents and, consciously or subconsciously, choose the bits we think they did well and carry them forward while simultaneously casting aside the areas we now identify as unhelpful or particular attributes that we want our own children to avoid being exposed to. In a few decades, we may well find ourselves being critically appraised by our own children about how we performed as parents, so it's worth giving careful consideration to the type of dad you want to become.

As I hold my burping bundle of daughter in my arms and try hard to assess whether she needs a nappy change or whether my nose has just become paranoid, I think about how much life has changed since her arrival. No matter how resolute I was in my thinking that having a baby 'wouldn't change me', it most certainly has. I had a self-centred approach to life, now I prioritize the happiness and welfare of my child and her other incredible carer, my wife. The love is so strong and the admiration so great that I'm constantly surprised by how these feelings continue to grow each day. When I'm exhausted, stressed about work or contemplating life's next steps, I can now look at the other two members of my family team and feel that, whatever life brings, as long as they're by my side, life will be good. I sometimes wonder what my children might say about me in a speech at my 60th birthday party or, more morbidly, what they might tell others about me when I'm no longer around. Children come into the world without preconception or prejudice and, as their dads, we're given a unique opportunity to inform, nurture, cherish and love them. I don't know how long I'll have to write the script of those speeches they'll give in years to come, but what I do know is that my time starts now.

What Women Want

DO accept any offers of babysitting, even if just to give you both a break for an hour to spend some quality time together.

DON'T forget to enjoy the early weeks; they're incredibly precious and will be gone before you know it.

Index

Acknowledgements

Unmeasurable thanks go to so many. My incredible wife, Rachel, for her unfaltering support throughout this process, her immaculate attention to grammar and her expert guidance in keeping me balanced somewhere between transparent and oversharing. Her skill at life makes her the perfect partner, whether parenting or otherwise, and this book would literally not have been possible without her warmth, love and ovaries. Thanks for bringing me doughnuts at the hardest times. Aurora, this is your story - or at least the very beginning of it. Your smile, attempts at typing and the daily joy you bring has inspired me to hopefully support other dads as they too embark on fatherhood. When you can one day read this, know that your dad loves you more than he could ever write in these pages. To Mum and Dad, for giving me the greatest start anyone could ever have hoped for in life and for never quashing my crazy ideas; you have been my rocks throughout. To all of my family and friends who've been so politely bored to tears by book concept ideas, cover design options and title choices.

To all of the team at John Noel Management, particularly Jonny Wilkinson for sharing the vision for this book and making it a reality, and of course to big John Noel himself. To all of the wonderful people at Octopus Publishing and Kyle Books, but especially Judith Hannam for trusting a doctor and tired new dad with a book contract and Sophie Allen for her expert guidance and ability to sensor my medical brain to prevent this book from putting people off having children altogether. To Matt Chinworth for his exceptionally tasteful illustrative interpretation of the text, against all odds.

To all those who've supported and trained me throughout my medical career, including the calm guidance of Shuman Hussein. Particular thanks to Jo Maynard and Sunita Sharma for their wisdom and technical input into these pages. To all the midwives, nurses, health visitors, doctors, admin and support staff I've been so privileged to work alongside, but above all to the team that superbly supported me and Rae as we welcomed Rory into the world.

Finally, to the dads, patients and families who have so openly shared their stories - whether crying with laughter or sadness - to help me bring you this book. From you I have learnt more than I could ever have imagined.